The
DHEA
Breakthrough

STEPHEN CHERNISKE, M.S.

Ballantine Books
New York

Some material in this book previously appeared in The
Great Soup Diet by Stephen Cherniske and Dr. Kenneth J. Frank,
Guildford & Cross Publishers. Reproduced by permission. Material also
was taken from articles originally published by Ms. Fitness
magazine and the News America Syndicate.

http://www.randomhouse.com

Library of Congress Catalog Card Number: 97-92951

ISBN: 0-345-41391-1

Manufactured in the United States of America
First Ballantine Books Trade Edition: June 1997
10   9   8   7   6   5   4   3

To Deborah, my wife and best friend, and to our sons,
Daniel and Mikhail

Contents

Acknowledgments

I am particularly indebted to Cynthia Anderson for her editorial and writing assistance. Her literary and technical skill and her enthusiastic support and focused attention were absolutely essential for the completion of this project. Special thanks to Michael Bennett, Pharm.D., for many consultations and his invaluable contributions to Chapters 10 and 11, and to research assistant and dear friend Grace Malonai for believing and always being there.

Thanks to all the dedicated and forward-thinking researchers and clinicians who saw the promise of DHEA early on and had the courage to act, particularly Drs. Arthur Schwartz, Samuel Yen, Jesse Hanley, Michael Rosenbaum, Alan Gaby, Etienne-Emile Baulieu, Jonathan Wright, Murray Susser, and Maria Majewska. Special thanks to my colleague Kenneth J. Frank, M.D., for counsel and friendship as well as his uncommon insight and medical expertise, and to Ferdy Massimino, M.D., who has always been an inspiration and mentor.

My warmest gratitude to Robert Stricker, literary agent and confidant, who found the very best home for this manuscript. To those at Ballantine who understand the crossroads where society now stands and their willingness to direct the "traffic" of critical information. Publisher Clare Ferraro, Associate Publisher Cathy Repetti, Senior Publicist Marie Coolman, Vice President for West Coast Publicity Liz Williams, Assistant Publicist Kristina White, and Assistant Editor Betsy Flagler.

To the staff and management of the Santa Barbara Athletic Club, my workshop, yoga studio, and human performance "laboratory." Thanks especially to Joy DuMay, Ken Gilbert, Wendy Bronson, Alice Chouinard, and Diana Zapata.

And finally, eternal gratitude to my mother, who endured the chemistry sets, dissected frogs, and experiments throughout the house. To my sister, who always paved the way for me, and to my father, who gave me his very best.

Preface to the

Second Edition

Since publication of *The DHEA Breakthrough* in September 1996, I've had the opportunity to speak with hundreds of readers, by phone, fax, modem, radio and TV call-ins, and in person. On my last cross-country flight, the seat next to me was a revolving door of people wanting to share their stories and ask their questions. It's been an incredibly rewarding experience because events have turned out exactly as I predicted.

By that I mean that the people who read the book and followed the DHEA plan have experienced remarkable results. A mother of four in New Orleans told me that she was back in shape and down to her pre-childbirth weight after feeling beaten down for fifteen years. An airline pilot stopped drinking ten cups of coffee a day, saw his blood pressure drop to normal, and felt like a new man. A Los Angeles woman in her mid-forties started on the DHEA plan and in two months had dropped four dress sizes, got off antidepressants, and was feeling better than she had since high school. A 61-year-old man told me of going from impotence and depression to vitality and sexual vigor in ninety days. And the DHEA plan also gave his 92-year-old father a new lease on life.

One element was common to all of these experiences: a feeling of vitality and strength that made all the difference. As you read the following chapters, try not to treat the material simply as information. Take time to imagine what the benefits and blessings that I describe would mean for you in your life. That will make the book more meaningful, more motivating, and even more rewarding for you.

I am continually amazed at people's ability to make significant changes—at the resilience of the human body and mind. And the experience of writing this book has reinforced my belief that *anyone* can turn their life around.

Obviously, it's not as easy as just taking DHEA. You will be frequently reminded in the following pages that the breakthrough here is a *program*, not a pill. And that's precisely why it works so well. The "magic bullet" approach has *never* worked, but the DHEA plan *will*, and you can start to experience the benefits in a matter of days.

That means the DHEA plan is self-perpetuating. As your metabolic efficiency improves, you'll experience greater energy. With greater energy, you'll enjoy being more active. With activity, you'll gain fitness; and with fitness, strength. No one will be standing over you shaking a finger. Your motivation and your desire will naturally move you forward. You'll see what life is like on what I call the upward spiral.

Of course, I also predicted that DHEA would become a fad, and a trip to your local health food store will confirm that. You will find DHEA that has been micronized, emulsified, activated, pre-digested, and potentized. The good news is that this book will guide you through the maze of hype and hoopla to the simple, scientific truth.

And speaking of science, important research published since the first edition continues to support the careful strategy presented in *The DHEA Breakthrough*. In fact, a recent editorial in the prestigious *Journal of Clinical Endocrinology and Metabolism* states that: "Logic pleads in favor of oral administration of DHEA at a dose that provides so-called "young" DHEA levels in the blood."*

Every day we make choices, and the sum of those choices creates our life. I encourage you to consider that this book may be in your hands for a very good reason. *The DHEA Breakthrough* may provide the tools and information you need to create the kind of life you want . . . a long life filled with joy and the fulfillment of your highest goals. I look forward to hearing your success story.

Stephen Cherniske
Santa Barbara, February 1997
FAX (805) 957-2040
E-mail: veritas@mem.po.com

*Baulieu, Etienne-Emile. Dehydroepiandrosterone (DHEA): A Fountain of Youth? *Journal of Clinical Endocrinology and Metabolism* 1996: 1(9); 3147–51.

The
DHEA
Breakthrough

Introduction

In the pursuit of a healthy body the most valuable possession is an open mind. A cynical attitude is an obstacle to learning, but blind acceptance is just as bad. It leads ultimately to confusion, error, and disappointment. The purpose of this book is to give you the information and tools you need to reap the rewards of optimum health without being taken for a ride or endangering your health.

Right now you can walk into a health food store and obtain DHEA, a potent hormone with remarkable biological activity throughout the body and brain. In some stores there is a choice of capsules or tablets, and soon there will also be transdermal patches and even a spray. DHEA gum is now on the drawing board at more than one company. What's going on?

The store clerks will tell you that DHEA can help you live longer; increase your libido; lower your risk of heart disease, cancer, and diabetes; and make you feel twenty years younger. If you ask about safety, they'll tell you that it's completely natural.

At that point two thoughts should come to mind. First, there are plenty of all-natural substances that can kill you, and related to that, should you trust a person with no training in medicine or health science? Working in a health food store is no indication of expertise. Orderlies work in hospitals, but you wouldn't ask one of them to remove your appendix. So where can you go for accurate advice? After all, many of your friends are taking DHEA and reporting amazing benefits. If half the claims are true, this is something you don't want to miss.

Unfortunately, it is unlikely that your doctor will be up to date regarding DHEA. He or she may have measured DHEA in rare cases of suspected adrenal malfunction, but few physicians are aware of the explosion in worldwide research suggesting that DHEA may in fact do everything the sales clerk claimed it would.

The DHEA Breakthrough is intended to give you a balanced view, as safety is an important and frequently neglected issue. Even more important, this book is not about a pill but about a *plan*, an integrated approach to living longer and better. The DHEA Plan incorporates the recent explosion of research concerning DHEA into the framework of human history and gives you a specific course of action to achieve optimum health and longevity. I suggest you read this book carefully and share it with your doctor in order to make intelligent decisions. One thing is for certain: DHEA is not something you should ignore.

WHAT EXACTLY IS DHEA?

DHEA is an acronym for a hormone produced by your adrenal glands known as dehydroepiandrosterone (*de-hydro-epi-an-DROS-ter-own*). The fact that it is now a household word (at least in millions of American homes) is not all that surprising given the American psyche, the aging population, and what I call "health hype."

It seems that every year our consumer-oriented society comes up with two or three "amazing" discoveries that promise instant weight loss or perfect health, and the common feature is that they all work effortlessly. Of course, the next year produces a new crop of miracle cures, and the old ones are debunked or ignored in favor of something newer and better. I don't want this to happen with DHEA.

Pure DHEA tablets are now available in health food stores and by mail, accompanied by flashy brochures making wild claims. After years of research, however, I can tell you that DHEA is *not* just another fad. But if it is *treated* like a fad, hyped to the sky, sold like snake oil, and promoted by greed, we will end up losing something of great value and promise. Fads create problems. If a product such as DHEA is promoted by untrained and/or unethical people, consumers will use it unwisely and hurt themselves. Another danger is that manufacturers will dilute the purity and create mistrust in the marketplace. *The DHEA Breakthrough* is intended to help avoid those pitfalls.

DHEA RESEARCH HEATS UP

Like many biochemists, I've been intrigued by DHEA for more than a decade. For years I updated my files about every six months by adding twenty or thirty new studies from the worldwide medical and scientific literature. Now this update program is automatic. I simply log on to an international database, ask for all studies published since my last update, and go about my business. Later, when time permits, I go back and review the research, cross-referencing the material to the appropriate files. For example, if a study explores the effect of DHEA on cholesterol levels, I copy it to one of my files on heart disease.

Then, in January 1994, I noticed that this computer update was taking far too long. Thinking that something was wrong, I watched as more than 120 studies scrolled down my screen. Six months later there were 185 more, and six months after that there were 244. Suddenly DHEA research was getting very hot.

Throughout the 1970s and 1980s, however, medical researchers ignored DHEA for the same reason they neglected vitamin E. It just didn't fit into the prevailing paradigm defined by a century-old obsession with deficiency disease. Imagine the impact of discovering a deficiency disease. Thousands of people throughout the southern states were suffering from pellagra, and then someone figured out that it's caused by a lack of niacin. Bingo—the disease is gone within five years. Or consider the discovery that a little thiamine can prevent beriberi. These breakthroughs created heroes and a mind-set that said that if a substance was *really* important, a lack of it should cause a disease.

But a lack of vitamin E or DHEA will not cause a visible disease. It may cause all manner of *invisible* health problems such as atherosclerosis, but we are only now making these correlations. In fact, we now know that supplementing with 100 to 400 IU of vitamin E can reduce the risk of heart disease by about 40 percent. Nevertheless, the U.S. Food and Nutrition Board still maintains the Recommended

Daily Allowance (RDA) at a paltry 15 IU, and one of the primary reasons cited is the lack of a deficiency disease.

And so it was with DHEA. Even though it is the most abundant steroid hormone produced in the human body, even though its age-related decline is unparalleled in human biochemistry, this decline does not produce a visible disease, and so, the thinking goes, how important can it be?

I will present evidence that the body's decline in DHEA production does in fact produce a very well known disease called death. In fact, declining production of DHEA may be a genetic trigger for the aging process both as an effect and as a contributing cause of senescence. The reason it took so long to figure this out is that DHEA, like vitamin E, has a wide range of activity. It's not localized in one particular tissue, nor does it have one specific receptor site. DHEA is everywhere in the human body, so researchers could not see the forest for the trees.

A LANDMARK CONFERENCE

But then all that changed. In the 1990s research on DHEA exploded around the world as scientists discovered correlations between DHEA and scores of diseases. A landmark conference sponsored by the prestigious New York Academy of Sciences in 1995 brought many of these exciting studies into the public spotlight. Even the name of the conference, "DHEA and Aging," had a provocative ring, and soon everyone was talking about the new wonder drug.

Looking at the conference program, I knew what was about to happen. I'd seen far lesser substances turn into overnight fads through a combination of media hype and industry hoopla. Here was a biochemical with extraordinary promise, backed for once by solid science. Presenters talked about DHEA's effect on immunity, aging, energetics, brain biochemistry, mind, mood, and behavior. But unlike the many other conferences I've attended, everyone there was making efforts to *downplay* his or her remarkable findings. Beyond the professional restraint that is expected of a scientist, it was perhaps the shared feeling that all this extraordinary news was just too good to be true. One group stated this clearly:

We must be skeptical of a single steroid that can cause weight loss in obese animals, correct blood sugar concentration in diabetic animals, decrease blood cholesterol, prevent athero-sclerosis, enhance the activity of the immune system, depress tumor formation, and improve the memory of aged mice.[1]

Something else was new at this conference: an obvious media presence. Reporters and camerapersons roamed the halls looking for a scoop, but the scientists typically responded with the disclaimer that their research was preliminary. More studies were needed. No recom-mendations for human use of DHEA could be made.

This, of course, was a lie. What they meant was that no *public* rec-ommendations could be made. The silent secret at that conference was that many of the presenters were taking DHEA themselves. I know this because I was a member of that small fraternity, and I shared news of the biochemical's effects with a number of colleagues across the nation. In fact, we often joked about how researchers invariably ended up purchasing additional DHEA for "future studies."

That a scientist would eagerly experiment on himself or herself with a powerful hormone is understandable once you read some of the research presented at this conference: studies showing that DHEA dramatically decreases the risk of heart disease, diabetes, osteoporosis, and cancer; extends the life span of animals up to 50 percent; enhances sexual function; cures impotence; and boosts memory and cognition. The antiobesity effects were some of the best news. DHEA is not simply an appetite suppressant; studies were showing that it alters metabolism to accelerate fat burning and foster gains in muscle mass. I would have been surprised if anyone involved in these break-through studies was *not* taking the drug.

By the conference's end we were all keenly aware that the genie had been let out of the bottle and that some level of control had to be placed on the media. That is when the party line was developed in which reporters were told that DHEA was a controlled substance available by prescription from only a few special compounding phar-macies.

In reality, we all knew doctors who were handing out prescrip-tions as fast as they could write them. We knew that there was a

growing "gray market" in DHEA, that AIDS and chronic fatigue patients were buying it from their support groups, and that it was the hot topic in locker rooms across the nation. Every week, it seemed, more and more people were talking about DHEA, and that worried me.

THE ROLE OF DHEA

You see, I believe that DHEA can play an extraordinary role in health and wellness, but I also know that the popular press and the health industry tend to oversimplify issues. They ignore the complexities of human physiology in order to package the next fad as a neat and easily consumed commodity. It happened with melatonin. Here is a hormone produced in microgram amounts by the pineal gland, and millions of Americans are now taking a hundred times that amount every day in a pill. No one knows what long-term effects overdosing with melatonin will have on the pineal gland. After all, high-dose intake of other hormones usually produces some suppression of glandular function, and some melatonin users are now experiencing symptoms of depression and short-term memory loss. It may be that the nutrition industry jumped the gun with melatonin.

It would be a tragedy if DHEA became the next craze. To prevent this, many of my colleagues are asking the U.S. Food and Drug Administration (FDA) to ban the substance, but I strongly disagree. Banning it would not prevent people from obtaining DHEA. It would only drive earnest and law-abiding citizens into a black market where purity and potency are unknown. Instead, I support efforts to provide accurate and balanced information that will enable men and women, with the help of their doctors, to make an informed choice.

Advertisements are now appearing in popular magazines, touting the wonders of DHEA. This is not informed choice. I can find DHEA in any number of health food stores, enthusiastically promoted by salesclerks, and articles are appearing on the Internet, written by people with little understanding of biochemistry or physiology. When I log on to request scientific support for their claims, only studies on rats or mice are provided. This is not informed choice, either. More human studies need to be done before the effects of DHEA are truly known.

STRIKING A BALANCE

In this book I strive to present a balanced point of view—an in-depth but easy-to-understand look at this remarkable biochemical—so that health-conscious individuals can take advantage of the breakthrough without hurting themselves. In addition, I hope that it will serve as a guide to clinicians beset by patients looking for a "fountain of youth" pill.

It's important to understand that there is no fountain of youth pill, but for twenty-five years, I have been telling my students and clients that there is a fountain of youth *lifestyle*. After all, the human body is designed to last about 120 years, and with proper care they can all be vibrantly healthy years. What DHEA provides is the missing link in your longevity program. It gives you a better-than-fighting chance against the diseases that cause more than 75 percent of premature deaths.

Think about that. We all know people who were healthy and robust until they got cancer. We've all read stories about incredibly fit men who went jogging one morning and ended up facedown on the sidewalk, dead from a heart attack. DHEA is a powerful anticancer and cardioprotective agent. That fact alone makes it worthwhile to safeguard its use. But there's much more. DHEA can make your later years energetic and passionate, as opposed to the progressive decrepitude most people experience. That's because it can help make you fit again.

That last sentence may turn off a lot of people, because fitness implies exercise and most people flee from exercise, not necessarily because they are lazy. I have found in more than a decade of clinical practice that most people hate exercise because it just makes them feel bad.

I've seen it a thousand times. People stop moving in their late twenties when they start a career. They may exercise sporadically, but it's not consistent enough to prevent the deconditioning of their muscles and metabolism. Then one day they look in the mirror and decide they have to "get in shape." Sound familiar? So they go to the gym or buy a video and try to follow the incredibly fit instructor, only to become exhausted halfway through the class. The next day every muscle aches. This is not exactly positive feedback, so it takes an incredibly strong person to go out and do that all over again. If you are incredibly motivated, you will make it through this period known as adaptation, but eight of ten people will quit before their bodies figure out where to get the extra energy that exercise requires.

It's a classic catch-22. You can't experience the exuberance and invigoration of exercise until you are fit, but you cannot get fit until you exercise consistently. It's the twentieth-century American dilemma, and because of that we have become the fattest and most unfit nation in history.

But what if I told you that you could reduce or completely eliminate the dreaded adaptation period, that there is now a way to increase your metabolic efficiency to the point where exercise becomes easier and more enjoyable? And what if that exercise produced rapid and visible rewards, the kinds of effects you remember as a teenager? Would you be willing to give that a try? If your answer is yes, this book is for you.

THE DHEA PLAN

Now, these benefits come not from a pill but from a plan. There's work involved, but unlike your past efforts, the DHEA Plan utilizes exercise that is *self-paced and moderate*. What's more, this plan will make you feel twenty years younger in a remarkably short period. It will change your life in countless ways and lead you to a new experience of vitality and health. By the way, that includes what I call nonobsessive weight management. Weight loss on the DHEA Plan is a by-product, a side effect, not the focus on the plan. It happens automatically without your becoming preoccupied with fat grams, calories, and appetite suppressants.

No matter where you are right now, the DHEA Plan can help get you back on the upward spiral. That's where you experience greater energy, so you naturally start to move. You exercise a little and feel better. You feel better, so your self-esteem improves. You start to take better care of yourself and make better nutritional choices, and that contributes to a greater feeling of energy, vitality, and health. Your friends and even your doctor want to know what you're doing. Your relationships improve, and life is transformed. And it all starts with the few simple changes presented in the chapters that follow.

ROOTS OF THE DHEA PLAN

It's important for you to know that the DHEA Plan was not pulled out of a hat. I'm a biochemist, but research occupies only part of my time. I'm really in the business of helping people fulfill their dreams. A few years ago a physician came to my office and told me his dream was to win a national triathlon championship. That's a reasonable goal for an extremely fit twenty-year-old, but this guy was thirty-three and a busy doctor. Nevertheless, he crossed the finish line in first place.

I've worked with members of the U.S. Olympic track and field team, and I've coached world record holders in mountaineering and martial arts. But more important than that is what has happened to thousands of people who just wanted to get through the day, people who found themselves in a downward spiral and didn't know how to turn it around. The DHEA Plan is the shortest and most reliable route to optimum health I've ever found, but still I am asked every day if there is a shortcut. This is because the American psyche is locked into an instant-results, no-think, no-move mind-set. So while there will be numerous books, hundreds of articles, and countless ads all promising that you can sit on your couch, watch TV, take DHEA, and live forever, it won't happen. That's the lie that got us into this mess in the first place.

The average life expectancy of an American is currently seventy-four years. It could be much longer, but we make dumb mistakes, we refuse to move, and we've been conditioned to accept a measly seventy-four-year life span. I accepted it, too, until my first biology course, when I discovered that the body is a miraculous self-repairing organism.

I learned that we have tremendous organ reserves that enable us to live far beyond 100 years. For example, your liver (if you do not overconsume alcohol) can do its present job quite well with one-third of its mass. You have more than you need. You can live quite happily with one kidney, but you have two. A man needs only one testicle, a woman only one ovary. Everywhere you look in the human body, you see backup systems to enhance our chances of living a very long time.

Then I came across immortal cell line research, in which scientists keep entire tissues alive, presumably forever, simply by providing essential raw materials and efficiently removing toxins and waste. That is what our circulatory and respiratory systems are designed to do, but as I said, we make dumb mistakes. We clog our arteries with fat, we breathe polluted air, and some of us intentionally inhale carcinogenic agents deep into our lungs. To make matters worse, the one activity that keeps both of these life support systems in shape is something we've decided we can do without: exercise. Today 60 percent of American adults are completely sedentary—that is, having no regular exercise in their lives.

MORE THAN A PLAN—A LIFESTYLE CHOICE

Our bodies are designed to move, but we lead sedentary lives. We are designed to consume a wide variety of fresh raw foods, but our diet is processed, refined, cooked, and chemicalized. We're stressed and burned out, and we live only seventy-four years. You can't fix all that just by taking DHEA. There needs to be a fundamental change in the way we look at life and the aging process.

This reevaluation includes modern medicine, where "progress" is primarily cut and paste. Sure, we can rip out a few arteries from a guy's leg and graft them into his heart, but is that a sensible way to manage heart disease? How about preventing the disease in the first place? We've got an arsenal of surgical and chemical weapons to fight the late stages of cancer, but what about *preventing* cancer or dealing with it at an earlier stage with nontoxic therapies?

All this is now possible with the help of DHEA, but DHEA alone is not enough. You cannot continue smoking cigarettes and benefit much from DHEA. You cannot live a sedentary life and expect to see fabulous results from DHEA. And you cannot eat junk or let your stress levels go through the roof and expect DHEA to repair the damage. But if you have decided that life is precious and you want more than a measly seventy-four years, please read on. The DHEA Plan will turn back the clock on a number of important metabolic factors that influence how fast your body ages. In other words, it is now possible not only to age slower but to enjoy greater energy and vitality, fewer illnesses, and greater mental clarity. Who could ask for more?

CHAPTER 1

Foundations
of the
DHEA Plan

My motto is, "If people knew better, they'd do better." And knowing does not mean simply reading or hearing information. There are plenty of books that provide a great deal of information on aging, but human beings are not motivated by information. We may be interested and entertained, but we are rarely moved to act. If information were powerfully motivating, no one would smoke cigarettes. And advice in the form of "shoulds" and "oughts" is the least effective type of information. Studies show that we tend to resent being told what to do. Perhaps it reminds us too much of our parents.

THE AWARENESS FACTOR

I learned about human resistance to information as a university instructor. I was paid to provide information, but I'm sure you noticed that teachers who merely fulfilled that requirement didn't exactly light your fire. Think about it. Which teachers inspired you to change your point of view or change your life? They were the ones who provided more than information: They increased *awareness*. Awareness is powerfully motivating. It can change everything in the blink of an eye, and that's what I worked at with my students. If I could present information in a way that increased awareness, I knew I would succeed. Because in teaching people how their bodies work, the goal is not just to inform but to help them live long, healthy, and joy-filled lives.

Take anatomy and physiology. There are plenty of good textbooks that present the facts, but why is it that students in general hate the class? After all, there is no subject more inspiring than the miraculous structure and function of life itself. But if the class is reduced to information, lists of organs and bones to memorize, it becomes a dreaded experience. That's a tragedy. Students miss out on a chance to gain awareness.

I developed what I called the "Anatomy Academy" approach to teaching these subjects. Long before the availability of computer animation and multimedia, I would have minimally clad volunteers (men and women) act as living models. As I talked about the astounding function of a particular muscle group, I would use water-based magic markers to identify it on a model. The words became action as the volunteer performed a particular movement. Joints and bones came to life in a similar way. And it worked. No one had trouble remembering where the spleen was or how the forearm bones accommodate the twisting of the hand.

I've spent a career making life science understandable and inspiring, but I've never tried to make it romantic. From a scientific point of view life is not romantic at all, and by that I mean that things happen the way they are designed to happen, not as we would wish them to. Americans have a hard time accepting that. That's why all Hollywood movies have happy endings. We just can't seem to understand that life does not conform to our desires until we are face-to-face with illness or the frightening experience of growing old.

THE DNA BLUEPRINT

Perhaps it is because Americans have developed such incredible technological powers that we assume that these powers of control extend to the functioning of our bodies. But in truth you are controlled by DNA, the microscopic strand of genetic material that lies deep within the nuclei of all your cells. We think we live in the "information age," but all the information your body will ever need is contained in your genes, strung onto chromosomes like beads on a necklace. It's all there: detailed instructions for millions of functions performed by trillions of cells, the immeasurably complex and miraculous process of life.

DNA also contains every characteristic that makes you who you are, every trait that you will pass on to future generations, and, most important, the accumulated wisdom of millions of years of human evolution. You may already know that on an intellectual level, but here's something to change your awareness. The ancient blueprint that controls every cell of your body hasn't changed at all—*not a fraction of 1 percent*—in more than twenty thousand years.

Of course, everything else has changed. And those changes have occurred very recently. To understand this, picture recent human evolution laid out on a timeline the length of a football field. You're standing at the end that represents today. At the opposite end stands a fellow who differs radically from the stereotypical "ape-man." He's standing quite straight, he has a brain almost as large as yours, and he knows how to make tools and use fire. He is *Homo sapiens*, and the point where he is standing represents 300,000 years ago.

Now, looking down the field, you have to understand that during the vast majority of that time nothing changed at all. The seasons changed, eons came and went, and humankind gradually accumulated more survival skills. Finally, at a point just past your three-yard line, we learned to grow food. At about the two-and-a-half-yard line we domesticated animals. But the industrial revolution is only 8 inches from your foot. Imagine the changes that have occurred in that incredibly short period of time. All the rest, 97 percent of the football field, represents the time humans spent as hunters and gatherers, the tail end of an era that actually lasted 1.6 million years. Paleolithic, very primitive times.

THE PALEOLITHIC PERSPECTIVE

There is no way our bodies could possibly have adapted to the astounding changes that have occurred in the last five thousand years, let alone the last five hundred years. We are in fact still tuned to the foods, conditions, activities, and behaviors of the ancient past, but we live in a time warp where everything is different.

Our gastrointestinal tract is designed for grazing, whereas today we gorge. For 1.6 million years, whenever we became hungry, we simply picked something and ate it, and we stopped eating as soon as our hunger was satisfied. Today we postpone hunger satisfaction to preset times called meals, during which we consume enormous amounts of food. Few of us stop when our hunger is gone; we eat until we're "full."

For 1.6 million years, when the sun went down, we went to sleep. Then, in 1879, the electric lightbulb was invented and all that changed. In the town where I live you can wash your clothes, go grocery shopping, bank, and watch TV twenty-four hours a day.

We seem to think that sleep is a waste of time when in reality it is incredibly important "down time" when the body is restored and repaired. And it's not just the body but the mind as well. Sleep keeps us sane, and the lack of sleep causes a great deal of mental and emotional dysfunction. Sleep research has shown that you can produce classic signs of psychosis in a person simply by disrupting his or her sleep three nights in a row. Mood, mind, and behavior are powerfully linked not only to the amount of sleep but to the quality of sleep. That brings up another point.

HABITAT DYSFUNCTION SYNDROME

For 1.6 million years we rested in the sounds of nature—a running stream, chirping crickets, singing birds—what are called primordial sounds. They are literally encoded in our genes, so it's no surprise that listening to these sounds today will lower your heart rate and blood pressure and put you at ease. By contrast, listening to police sirens, traffic noise, and television violence produces anxiety and contributes to illness.

In college I helped care for the monkeys and chimpanzees in the primate lab, and we had a 4-inch-thick manual that listed their habitat characteristics in minute detail. That was the book we went to whenever they got sick or upset, and the amazing thing was that their illness or distress was usually resolved by adjusting the lab conditions to match their natural habitat more closely.

Anyone who has been around chimps will tell you that they're just like children. And since fathering children of my own, I have come to formulate what I call the *habitat dysfunction syndrome*. You see, I don't have a habitat manual for my kids. When they get sick or upset, my wife and I do the best we can, and sometimes we take them to the doctor. But I always wonder what children would be like if they were living in their natural habitat, eating purely natural foods, exposed only to the full-spectrum light of the sun and the verdant greens, earthy browns, and bright blue colors of nature.

We all suffer to some degree from habitat dysfunction syndrome, depending on how we live. I try to live as close to nature as possible, not because I'm a "health nut" but because I know that 98.4 percent of my genes are exactly the same as those of chimps. That's right: The difference between you and a chimpanzee is 1.6 percent of your DNA. Makes you think, because we are so far removed from our natural habitat that it is impossible to evaluate the harm we suffer as a result.

When was the last time you walked through a dense tropical forest? I remember the experience vividly because of the way it made me feel: relaxed, incredibly alive, and free. Whenever I'm in a forest, I feel great, whether it's in the Everglades or the California redwoods. Then I look at data showing that the incidence of cancer increases the farther you live from the equator. I look at the crime rate in our crowded cities or data showing that mental illness increases in direct proportion to population density, and none of that surprises me. It's habitat dysfunction syndrome. Our technology has outstripped our biology.

There is no area of science where this time warp does not factor in heavily, and I am convinced that it is the key to the quest for health and wellness. We can't go back to Paleolithic times, and who would want to? The point is that *awareness* of our modern predicament, the fact that we are literally out of sync with our genes, opens the door to understanding how to use technology, information, and today's remarkable biochemicals to our greatest benefit.

CAVE MEN IN SUITS

When I am sitting in a 747, flying at 580 miles an hour, typing on my laptop computer, and talking on the phone, I remind myself that I am a caveman dressed in a suit. My brain understands all this technology, but my body does not.

People often suffer from serious circulation problems caused by sitting too long. Not me. Whether traveling or sitting at my desk, I make sure to move my Paleolithic body for ten minutes at least every two hours. I stretch, walk up three flights of stairs, do push-ups or knee lifts. On airplanes I'm the guy sitting in the bulkhead seat with his feet high against the wall. During stopovers I do yoga or tai chi. I get three vegetarian lunches and graze for hours. Call me crazy, but it works.

The Paleolithic perspective is a tremendous advantage in the quest for optimum health whether you want to lose weight, maximize your life span, have more energy, enjoy deeper and more restoring sleep, improve your memory, boost your immunity, or all of the above. It is the foundation awareness that I'll refer to in every chapter of this book, because it is the silent force encoded in your genes.

EVOLUTION: A PROGRAM FOR SURVIVAL

You might not know that Paleolithic men and women were healthier, stronger, and even taller than people in many modern societies. Sure, we have a higher overall life expectancy today, but if a hunter-gatherer made it to age sixty, her chances of seeing ninety were just as good as yours. The point is that we now have the opportunity to sur-pass anything that has ever gone before as long as we don't forget where we came from.

I am surprised at the lack of attention paid to evolution by longevity researchers. It seems that in looking ahead, many have for-gotten the past. And the most important point for any researcher to remember, whether he is looking at plants, reptiles, birds, primates, or any other living thing, is this: The sole purpose of every system, tissue, gland, organ, and hormone is *survival*.

Imagine you are an evolutionary biologist and you can begin to understand the depth of this truth. When others wonder why diets fail, you know that the ability to store fat was perhaps the most impor-tant evolutionary development that enabled humankind to survive. You see that conventional weight-loss diets only duplicate an ancient hazard (famine) and produce the same survival response (decreased metabolic rate and increased fat storage). Thus, people who diet tend to gain weight. Their bodies are simply doing what human bodies have done for 1.6 million years.

Others wonder why women tend to store fat more easily than men do. You know that it's another survival mechanism. After all, once a sperm fertilized the egg, the man (evolutionarily speaking) was expendable, but the woman had to nourish a baby until it could find food for itself.

Most people are surprised (and no doubt dismayed) to learn that our bodies and brains are controlled by twenty-thousand-year-old DNA. That understanding changes everything. It explains why women (often subconsciously) place a high emphasis on fitness in choosing a mate. There is an ancient awareness embedded in the primitive part of a woman's brain that says, "This man can help me survive."

In measuring the activity of a baby's brain, what do you think causes the greatest stimulation—receiving a favorite toy or seeing Mommy and Daddy kiss? It's the kiss. Why? Because the infant may love the toy, but that's only entertainment. Seeing Mommy and Daddy kiss tells the baby that this guy (Daddy) is going to stick around and help them survive. Likewise, new parents often report an enhanced attraction to each other. This is due to biochemicals known as *pheromones* that are produced by our brains and bodies to assure the survival of the infant.

Now, how does all this relate to DHEA? To understand that, we have to look at what DHEA does. It's an exciting story.

THE FIRST DHEA BREAKTHROUGH

Think back to *Homo sapiens* at the end of the football field. Remarkably, one of the evolutionary developments that got him there was the ability to produce DHEA—*lots* of DHEA. In fact, it's one of the most significant factors that separated him from the other animals, because brain growth requires an extraordinary amount of DHEA.

No one knows how or exactly when primates performed this biochemical feat, but *Homo sapiens* more than likely owed her ingenuity for tool making and ultimately language and technology to the intricate workings of DHEA and natural selection. As a result, you and I are here today, figuring out how to use the same substance not only to survive but to enjoy a long, happy, and fulfilling life. It's an opportunity that is, of course, quite new in the scheme of human history and one we should never take for granted.

DHEA IN OUR BODIES

When our adrenal glands produce DHEA, most of the hormone is stabilized as DHEA sulfate (DHEAS). DHEAS is then converted and metabolized to a number of other hormones, most notably but not limited to the sex hormones testosterone and estrogen.

The singular importance of DHEA is illustrated by the fact that approximately 50 percent of total androgens (male hormones) in adult men are derived from DHEA. In women the best estimates are that DHEA contributes perhaps 70 percent of estrogens before menopause and close to 100 percent afterward.

And it's not just about sex hormones. Researchers are finding DHEA receptors (biochemical trigger sites) on immune cells and on a wide variety of tissues throughout the body. We are only beginning to uncover the vast contribution of DHEA to human health.

What is startling is that our production of DHEA decreases markedly with age. After peaking at around age twenty-five, DHEA drops steadily in both men and women. Importantly, it is the only hormone in the human body that decreases in this dramatic fashion, making it a reliable marker of aging. By age seventy-five, blood levels of DHEAS in many people have dropped 95 percent from what I call "prime peak."

DHEA DECLINE AND DEATH: CAUSE AND EFFECT?

Put on your evolutionary biologist hat and look at the following chart. You know that in mammals, levels of DHEA correlate directly with average life span. You know that DHEA is the precursor to many other vitally important hormones, especially sex hormones. Your colleagues are telling you that DHEA is critically important to immune function, brain biochemistry, cardiovascular health, and the maintenance of muscle and bone. You're intrigued by the steep decline in DHEA that bottoms at around age seventy-five. Then you remember that the present life span is around seventy-five, and you start to put two and two together. What is your revelation?

Right! You postulate that there may be a cause-and-effect relationship between the declining production of DHEA and death. But

DECLINE IN DHEAS LEVELS WITH ADVANCING AGE

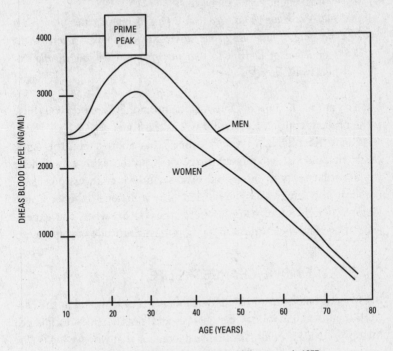

Adapted from Orentreich, et al., 1984, and Migeon, et al., 1957.

what is the *nature* of that relationship? That's the sizzle in this whole line of inquiry, and here's your reasoning:

GIVEN: The only function of a hormone (or any biochemical) is survival.

GIVEN: Survival of the *species* is the primary concern. Survival of the individual is important only insofar as it helps ensure survival of the species. Cold but true.

THUS: A hormone essential to reproductive function tends to peak when the organism is healthy and strong.

THUS: This hormone will decline when the organism is past its prime.

THUS (and here's where it gets interesting): It may be that the decline of this hormone is not an effect of aging but an actual *cause.* The ancient message embedded in our genes, in other words, might very well be this:

DNA to brain: This organism is past its reproductive prime. It is therefore of little use to the survival of the species. Decrease the production of DHEA so that the organism will die in approximately five decades.

You are the organism. DHEA is the hormone. What do you think is the prudent course of action for you at this time?

Right! Keep DHEA levels at prime peak. Short-circuit this aging clock, this ticking evolutionary time bomb, so that your cells believe you are still twenty-five years old. And see how it changes your life—not only the length of your life but also your level of energy and vitality. Watch the cascade of effects that occurs when you experience at age fifty the enthusiasm and optimistic attitude of your youth.

CHANGE THE MOVIE, CHANGE THE LIFE

Everyone is talking about the physical benefits of DHEA, but the psychological and emotional benefits should not be underestimated. Medical science is finally starting to document that who we are is to a great extent determined by what we think and how we *feel*. Over the years, in other words, we tend to outpicture what our minds project. That is the conclusion of antidepressant research: the concept of a vicious cycle in which the individual is simply fulfilling a self-negating mind movie. Change the movie, change the life.

With the DHEA Plan we are doing a great deal more because you're changing not just your attitude but your physical and mental ability as well. Imagine having the enthusiastic outlook of your youth, together with improved metabolic efficiency, so that exercise becomes easier and more enjoyable. Imagine having improved memory and cognition skills at an age when your parents were starting to forget names and lose car keys. *All this is now possible.*

I have had clients who started feeling these benefits and stopped the program. Some genuinely felt that there was something ethically wrong with turning back the clock. I would argue that all we are doing is maximizing the quality and quantity of life by optimizing or in some cases supplementing the body's naturally produced resources. Some people, however, can't accept that. They don't think they *deserve* to feel or look that good, and there's no counterargument for that. But if you've read this far, I suspect you wouldn't mind feeling and looking twenty years younger.

THE ROAD AHEAD

What would be the consequence of 72 million baby boomers with prime peak levels of DHEA? It's entirely possible, and I suggest that it will be a turning point for humankind. For the first time in history a great many men and women will be able to fulfill their most cherished dreams, and that makes for a healthy society.

I've always lamented the cruel irony of life: Just when knowledge and wisdom blossom in maturity, our capabilities start to fade. I've seen it in my grandparents and my parents. My father finally developed the tolerance and love that would enable him to be happy, only to die a few short years later of cancer. My mother, now almost eighty, will not suffer the same fate. She learned the lessons of love, compassion, and service early in life during thirty years as a nurse. But she has also been able to take advantage of modern biochemistry. She's fit, active, healthy, and full of surprises.

Recently, when I phoned at my accustomed time and found my mother not home, I became concerned. I called her neighbor, who told me that her car was gone, so I continued calling every hour. When I finally reached her, she exclaimed, "Oh, I forgot to tell you; I'm volunteering at the hospital." "Doing what?" I asked. "Oh," she intoned happily, "I'm driving old people to their doctors' appointments."

THE PRESENT STATUS OF DHEA

More than four thousand scientific studies have been conducted with DHEA, but there is still no complete and reliable protocol for its use. That's because most of those studies were conducted with animals, not humans. The reason for this is peculiar, having to do with the politics and economics of medical research.

DHEA is technically an "orphan drug," meaning that it has no parent company to guide its development through various stages of animal and human research. Although a patent could be obtained for a formulation containing DHEA, no pharmaceutical company is willing to spend the tens of millions of dollars necessary for FDA approval, knowing that competitors (and even the over-the-counter distributors) could then use the research to market their own products.

In the meantime, all the research and early clinical news have created a tremendous demand for DHEA, and a 1994 act of Congress, the Dietary Supplement Health and Education Act (DSHEA), opened the door to over-the-counter distribution. This legislation made a distinction between nutritional supplements and drugs, containing terminology that has since been used to create a "gray area" for products such as melatonin and DHEA.

In other words, by defining nutritional supplements as substances of natural origin, or natural to the human body, one could make a case for DHEA as a nutritional supplement. After all, it is certainly a natural substance, being created by the adrenals from cholesterol, and cholesterol, of course, is a component of food. The argument is a bit strained, but so far the FDA has decided not to take action to remove DHEA from the market. In fact, the 1994 legislation stipulates that for the FDA to ban a substance, it must first show it to be unsafe.

The DEA (U.S. Drug Enforcement Agency) has also taken a long hard look at the substance because an argument could be made that DHEA is a sort of anabolic steroid. As you will see in the following chapters, DHEA can be converted to testosterone in the body, and it has definite anabolic (tissue-building) properties. But apparently the DEA has decided (I think wisely) that DHEA poses little danger compared with the powerful anabolic steroids commonly used by athletes and body builders. If a body builder wanted to bulk up in a hurry, massive doses of DHEA would probably provide disappointing results, as much of the substance would be converted to counterproductive estrogen hormones.

From my perspective, there are both advantages and disadvantages to DHEA's current status.

Advantages

1. **AVAILABILITY.** I think it is extremely valuable to have DHEA available today, not in ten or fifteen years when confirming studies

have been conducted and mountains of red tape have been overcome. If you are twenty years old, you have the luxury of waiting, but there are 25 million baby boomers out there and all their parents who can benefit right now. I believe that there is more than enough research available to establish safety at low to moderate doses of 10 to 50 mg per day.

2. PRICE. A ninety-count bottle of 25 mg tablets costs about $15 in a health food store. I would venture to say that if DHEA were a prescription drug, you would have to pay three to four times that amount. When the substance was available only through compounding pharmacies, ninety tablets cost approximately $100.

3. EXPANDED RESEARCH. When no single corporation or entity is in control, there is a better chance that a substance will be thoroughly and completely researched and that all its potential benefits will be explored.

Disadvantages

1. Industry hype will tend to create a DHEA fad. People will expect miracles, and when they do not get instant results, many will increase the dose, believing that more is better. However, until more research is done with humans and DHEA, a physiologic dose of 10 to 50 mg is your safest bet.

2. Purity and potency are not closely monitored in the nutrition supplement industry, which is not to say they can't be improved. If consumers demand exceptional quality controls (outlined in Chapter 10), manufacturers will provide them.

3. I know many brilliant researchers who are eager to get involved in DHEA research but are frustrated by the lack of funds. University and foundation grants typically are barely enough to cover animal experiments, and we already have enough of those. Besides, animals are not a good model of DHEA metabolism. Large-scale human studies need to be conducted as soon as possible.

CONCLUSION: EDUCATE, DON'T REGULATE

When it comes to DHEA, I say *educate, don't regulate*. And while I believe this book presents sufficient information for you to make an informed choice regarding DHEA use, I want to emphasize the need for guidance from a well-informed health care professional to maximize the benefits and minimize the potential problems.

Look at it this way. DHEA research is an arena that is evolving *by the day*. Your health food store manager is not tied into that research. All he or she gets are the promotional materials from the manufacturers. Your friends (unless they are astute researchers tapping into international data banks) are not tied into that research. But physicians have remarkable access to information regarding DHEA and related issues. And they don't have to be endocrinologists. With today's technology, any physician can educate himself or herself in an unbelievably short period of time.

Physicians' Online® (POL) was launched in 1996, and it is providing a remarkable free service to physicians. Not only does it access MEDLINE, CANCERLIT, and other invaluable databases, but there are ongoing discussion groups related to a wide variety of topics, including DHEA. Any physician who wants to get on-line can do so quite easily. It's no longer a matter of going to the medical library, finding a place to park, spending hours researching a few topics, spending more hours finding the issues of the journal you want, and losing income (no one pays a doctor to keep up to date).

All that has changed. In a matter of minutes a physician can now access scientific and medical literature and, with the click of a mouse, discuss that research with colleagues. In fact, these discussion groups often include the study authors. To make it even easier, there are services that will scan the medical literature on a specific topic and E-mail relevant abstracts on a monthly or weekly basis. This astounding technology is already revolutionizing medical education, and the benefits are easy to see.

Regarding funding, I believe strongly that the National Institute on Aging (NIA) or another federal research organization should underwrite extensive clinical evaluations. With the remarkable benefits from DHEA we have seen in animal studies and the preliminary work with humans, it would be a tragedy if research were not vigorously pursued. I encourage you to write your congressperson or the NIA to voice your support.

THE OPPORTUNITY OF A LIFETIME

We are standing on the threshold of a new era that will enable us to move beyond the constraints and limitations of evolution. I am not referring to the science-fiction promises of genetic engineers. They may solve the puzzle of hereditary disease, but they will not in the near future produce a longevity tool for the masses. That tool already exists, and it will be unfolded in the chapters of this book.

Many people are already using DHEA to enjoy longer, more energetic, more fulfilling, and pain-free lives. The message that they are sending to their cells is this: "Life is good. I am a powerful and positive contributor to the general welfare of humankind." And the message they are receiving back is profound: "Good for you. I think I'll keep you around." What are the possibilities of this new dialogue? No one knows, but I invite you to find out for yourself.

BIBLIOGRAPHY

Austad SN. Menopause: An evolutionary perspective. *Exp Gerontol* 1994; 29(3–4):255–63.

De Paretti E, Forest MG. Pattern of plasma DHEAS levels in humans from birth to adulthood: Evidence for testicular production. *J Clin Endocrinol Metab* 1978; 47:572–7.

De Paretti E, Forest MG. Unconjugated DHEA plasma levels in normal subjects from birth to adolescence in humans. *J Clin Endocrinol Metab* 1976; 43:982–90.

Dobzhansky T, et al. *Evolution.* San Francisco: Freeman, 1977.

Eaton SB. What did our late Paleolithic (preagricultural) ancestors eat? *Nutri Rev* 1990; 48(5):227–30.

Johnson C. *Introduction to Natural Selection.* Baltimore: University Park Press, 1976.

Labrie F, et al. DHEA and peripheral androgen and estrogen formation: Intracrinology. *Ann NY Acad Sci* 1995; 774:16–28.

Lopez A. Metabolic and endocrine factors in aging, in *Risk Factors for Senility.* H Rothschild (ed.). Oxford University Press, New York, 1984, 205–19.

Lutz W. [The carbohydrate theory]. *Wien Med Wochenschr* 1994; 144(16): 387–92.

Migeon CJ, Keller AR, Lawrence B, Shepard TH. Dehydroepiandrosterone and androsterone levels in human plasma: Effect of age and sex, day-to-day and diurnal variations. *J Clin Endocrinol Metab* 1957; 17:1051–62.

Orentreich N, Brind JL, Rizer RL, Vogelman JH. Age changes and sex differences in serum dehydroepiandrosterone sulfate concentrations throughout adulthood. *J Clin Endocrinol Metab* 1984; 59:551–5.

Ravaglia G, Forti P, Maioli F, Boschi F, Bernardi M, Pratelli L. The relationship of DHEAS to endocrine-metabolic parameters and functional status in the oldest old: Results from an Italian study on healthy free-living over-ninety-year-olds. *J Clin Endocrinol Metab* 1996; 81:1173–7.

Smith MR, Rudd BT, Shirley A, Rayner PH, Williams JW, Duighan NM, Bertrand PV. A radioimmunoassay for the estimation of serum dehydro-epiandrosterone sulfate in normal and pathological sera. *Clin Chlm Acta* 1975; 65:5–13.

CHAPTER 2

Sex

You may not agree with Freud that libido, or the sex drive, is the primary motivating force in human behavior. You may prefer to think that human beings are inspired by "higher" or purer desires, and of course we are. But the fact remains that libido is a powerful (if not *the* most powerful) drive that is hardwired into our genes. It's there on the conscious level and in the subconscious, and if you believe Freud, it rules the unconscious domain of our existence. The reason is obvious: survival of the species.

Thousands of volumes have been written over the centuries dealing with the so-called struggle that humans have with this "base" desire, but I'll leave that debate to the philosophers and theologians. Hedonists celebrate it, moralists try to control it, and Madison Avenue exploits it, but from a scientific point of view libido is simply part of our biochemical and behavioral makeup.

THE COMPLEXITIES OF LIBIDO

Libido is generated by a complex combination of hormones and is also profoundly affected by other nonhormonal factors, including overall health, bioenergetics, and a raft of psychological and emotional responses.

One myth about libido is that men make testosterone and women make estrogen. In reality, *both* men and women make *both* hormones, although in different quantities. Another myth is that the sex drive is a "testosterone thing." In fact, normal adults (both men and women) possess greatly varying levels of testosterone, but studies have shown no evidence that these variations alone account for differences in sexual drive or behavior. Other hormones, such as estrogen and prolactin, also play an influential role in sexual response.

THE THREE STAGES OF SEXUAL RESPONSE

Scientists have identified three stages of human sexual response: sexual desire, sexual arousal, and orgasm. Sexual desire and arousal are so closely related that even scientists find it difficult to determine where one ends and the other begins. Key factors in sexual desire include an individual's frequency of sexual thoughts and fantasies, level of interest in initiating sexual contact, awareness of sexual cues, and frustration from unfulfilled sexual desires. The arousal stage includes sensations of sexual excitement and pleasure, along with the appropriate physiological responses that ultimately culminate in the third stage—orgasm.

Because of its effects across the entire spectrum of personal health, the DHEA Plan optimizes all three stages of sexual response, leading to a healthy and robust sex drive. Just as important, it will help you generate the energy and vitality to fulfill your desires.

EXERCISE AND OTHER "SEX CUES"

We know that people who exercise regularly tend to have sex more often than do their sedentary peers, but what is it about exercise that can explain that? Perhaps it's not exercise at all but simply the fact that highly charged people tend to exercise and enjoy sex. Well, current research shows that there *is* a cause-and-effect relationship: Exercise produces hormonal, biochemical, and psychological changes that all tend to increase libido and enhance sexual pleasure.

Did you know that there are substances you can take that will do wonders to increase your energy level as well as make exercising easier and more enjoyable? In Chapter 6 you'll learn how to stoke your fires with this powerful group of substances known as *bioenergetic nutrients*.

Libido of course is not simply a matter of exercise and energy. Nature didn't take any chances and loaded every sensory system with sex cues. The sense of smell, for example, is a powerful influence on preferences and desires. Research shows that babies are naturally attracted to the smell characteristics of their mothers. Children are fond of sweet, fruity smells and are unimpressed or repelled by heavier scents.

But all that changes at puberty. Adolescent boys and girls suddenly become attracted to heavier earthy or animal scents such as musk and sandalwood. Musk is a constituent of the sexual attractants produced by many animal species. It's all part of nature's master plan to turn on our libido and get us to procreate.

MEET THE ANDROGEN FAMILY

Besides testosterone, libido researchers have identified important roles for other hormones in the androgen family, including DHEA, DHEAS, and androstenedione. Androgens appear to be particularly critical for the arousal stage of libido, having powerful effects on both the endocrine (hormonal) and neurological (mental and emotional) systems. What's more, we are learning that women need these factors just as much as men do, although in smaller amounts and not just to increase libido. A recent report in the *American Journal of Medicine* identified a disorder known as "female androgen deficiency syndrome," characterized by impaired sexual functioning, fatigue, depression, and headache. The authors of the report suggest that androgen supplementation may help.

> Androgen replacement therapy is a neglected area of medical practice and further research is needed to identify all women who will benefit from it since studies in menopausal women have shown [oral] administration to be well tolerated and safe. Such therapy is underused and very much underresearched.[1]

Enter DHEA. Research shows that women convert a significant amount of this androgen to testosterone and androstenedione and that DHEA provides a number of other benefits as well, including conversion in the skeleton to bone-preserving estrogens.

DHEA appears to be nature's all-purpose energizing sex and health hormone. The only problem is that our bodies run out of it too soon.

THE SANDS OF TIME

Unfortunately, as we age, both the desire for sex and the ability to enjoy sex diminish. Men have increasing difficulty achieving and maintaining erections, and after menopause women experience vaginal dryness, diminished interest in sex, and atrophy of the vaginal muscles. While some people see these developments as an inevitable part of life, others miss the intensity and excitement of sexual activity.

If you want to stay sexually active, I have good news. After raising DHEA levels, men often find that sexual performance improves. Many report that erections become stronger and that ejaculatory volume and force are increased. A fifty-five-year-old friend of mine was elated with the results that he experienced with 50 mg of DHEA per day. "It's not just the sex," he noted, "but the feeling of renewed vigor, waking up every morning with the flag flying."

Clinicians in general claim that female patients report increases in libido even more frequently than males do. This might be explained by the fact that DHEA supplementation (at moderate doses) appears to raise testosterone levels in women more than it does in men.

This brings up another interesting theory. Some researchers believe that DHEA was in part responsible for the crowning achievement of humankind: the divergence of hominids from other primates. While other primates engage in sex only during estrus, a higher level of testosterone (derived from DHEA) might have made it possible for women to engage in sex throughout the female cycle. This would have given our female ancestors a competitive advantage, which no doubt increased their reproductive rate and assured through natural selection the emergence of *Homo sapiens*.

But what can DHEA do for us today? The answer to that lies in the combination of modern biochemical knowledge and an awareness of our Paleolithic genetic inheritance. In other words, you and I know that the survival of the species is a certainty, at least in terms of successful reproduction, but our genes are still locked into a procreate-or-die mode.

THE DHEA PLEASURE PRINCIPLE

For the first time in the history of humankind it appears that we can extend our life span and at the same time extend our number of sexually active years. That way, we not only get to enjoy the pleasures of sex but at the same time send "youth" messages to our cells that may postpone senescence and death.

Once again, the idea is to convince our cellular DNA that we are capable of reproducing. As long as that is a possibility, research with animals suggests that we may be able to extend the life span by 20 to 50 percent. As the saying goes, "Use it or lose it."

It's not simply a matter of taking a DHEA pill. DHEA will not instantly turn a middle-aged man or woman into a sex machine, but as an integral part of a longevity and vitality program DHEA can make a tremendous difference, and it's far superior to any of the pharmaceutical options available today.

SEXUAL PERFORMANCE AND PRESCRIPTION DRUGS

Research on human sexuality has escalated in recent years partly because of the ever-increasing rate of sexual disorders and the role played by prescription drugs in sexual dysfunction. Men and women taking a wide range of prescription drugs commonly experience decreased libido, erectile dysfunction, ejaculation delay, and orgasmic dysfunction. The main offenders are antipsychotics, antidepressants, mood-stabilizing agents, minor tranquilizers, and hypotensives. See the following list and consult a medical professional if you suspect you have a problem.

DHEA VERSUS HUMAN GROWTH HORMONE

You may have heard about the experiments with human growth hormone (HGH) that hit the news in 1992. Elderly men and women receiving HGH injections experienced greater energy, increased

PRESCRIPTION DRUGS THAT CAN CAUSE SEXUAL DYSFUNCTION

Drugs Reported to Decrease Libido

Acetazolamide
Alpha-methyldopa
Alprazolam
Amitriptyline
Amoxapine
Chlorpromazine
Chlorthalidone
Cimetidine
Clofibrate
Clomipramine
Clonidine

Clorazepate
Diazepam
Dichlorphenamide
Digoxin
Fenfluramine
Fluphenazine
Guanethidine
Hydrochlorothiazide
Imipramine
Lithium
Methazolamide

Phenelzine
Phenobarbital
Primadone
Propranolol
Protriptyline
Reserpine
Spironolactone
Thioridazine
Thiothixine

Drugs Reported to Cause Arousal Difficulties

Alpha-methyldopa
Amitriptyline
Amoxapine
Bendrofluazide
Bethanidine
Chlorpromazine
Cimetidine
Clofibrate
Clomipramine
Clonidine
Desipramine
Digoxin
Disulfiram

Doxepin
Fluphenazine
Guanethidine
Guanoclor
Guanoxan
Haloperidol
Hydrochlorothiazide
Imipramine
Isocarboxazid
Ketamine
Lithium
Maprotiline
Nortriptyline

Perhexiline
Phenelzine
Pimozide
Propranolol
Protriptyline
Reserpine
Spironolactone
Sulpiride
Thiabendazole
Thioridazine
Thiothixine
Tranylcypromine
Trazodone

Drugs Reported to Cause Orgasm Disturbances

Alpha-methyldopa
Alprazolam
Amitriptyline
Amoxapine
Bethanidine
Chlorpromazine
Chlorprothixine
Chlordiazepoxide
Clomipramine
Desipramine
Doxepin

Fluphenazine
Fluoxetine
Guanethidine
Haloperidol
Imipramine
Isocarboxazid
Lorazepam
Maprotiline
Mesoridazine
Naproxen
Nortriptyline

Paroxetine
Perphenazine
Phenelzine
Protriptyline
Sertraline
Thioridazine
Thiothixine
Tranylcypromine
Trazodone
Trifluoperazine

Source: Schiavi R, Segraves R, The biology of sexual function. Psychiatr Clin North Am 1995; 18(1): 7–23.

muscle mass and strength, increased skin thickness, and overall feelings of well-being. The problem was that all those benefits disappeared when they stopped the injections.

So why stop? The treatments are extraordinarily expensive ($12,000 per year), require someone to administer the injection, and side effects are fairly common. In recent research, some men developed breast swelling, a condition known as gynecomastia. Since HGH stimulates the growth of connective tissue, carpal tunnel syndrome, a painful narrowing of the nerve channel in the wrist, was fairly common. Some people developed arthritis and abnormal joint growth. Others experienced fluid retention and blood sugar abnormalities. Today research on HGH is continuing, but the "fountain of youth" expectations have been largely discounted.

DHEA, by contrast, produces most of the same benefits without the inconvenience of injection, the side effects, or the expense. In fact, you will learn in Chapter 3 that the mechanism by which these two substances produce such favorable changes is exactly the same: stimulation of a biochemical called insulin-like growth factor-1 (IGF-1) that sends rebuild-and-restore messages throughout the body.

DHEA VERSUS TESTOSTERONE SUPPLEMENTS

A great deal of work is being done today to evaluate the effects and side effects of testosterone supplements in aging men, and the data are not conclusive. First, there is no age-related decline in testosterone as there is with DHEA. That means that contrary to what you might read in a men's magazine, there is no male menopause corresponding to a woman's midlife decrease in estrogen production. Men do experience significant biochemical and psychophysical changes, but those changes cannot be attributed to a dramatic decrease in testosterone. Studies show that sexual activity in men sixty-five to eighty years of age is not related to testosterone levels.

DHEA appears to have a wider spectrum of effects and benefits throughout the body than does testosterone. A high level of DHEA confers more than sex enhancement. Keeping blood levels of DHEA at or near prime peak appears to improve overall immunity, increase energy, decrease body fat, strengthen bones, and decrease the risk of heart disease and cancer. Testosterone can influence *some* of those factors, but there's the DHEA advantage.

SIDE EFFECTS OF TESTOSTERONE SUPPLEMENTS

Testosterone administration has three potentially dangerous side effects. First, it can increase the risk of cardiovascular disease. Second, there is the feedback loop between the bloodstream and the testes. When blood levels rise, the testes decrease testosterone production, and if enough testosterone is supplied from an exogenous (outside) source, the testes shrink and may even lose their functional ability.

As far as we know, no feedback loop exists between DHEA and the adrenals. The administration of other adrenal hormones, such as cortisol, will cause a decrease in adrenal production, but leading researchers agree that this does not appear to be the case with DHEA. It is possible that adrenal suppression occurs at extremely high doses, but that remains to be seen.

The third danger with testosterone supplements is the increased risk for abnormal prostate enlargement known as benign prostatic hypertrophy (BPH) and prostate cancer. BPH affects nearly all men as they age, causing discomfort and occasionally pain. Because the enlarged prostate presses against the urinary tract, BPH's primary symptom is the inability to void the bladder completely. This means frequent nocturnal wakings to urinate and the frustration of not being able to relieve urinary pressure. Abnormal growth of the prostate is directly related to the rate at which testosterone is converted to dihydrotestosterone. Herbs such as saw palmetto (*Serenoa repens*) and drugs such as finasteride interfere with this conversion and slow down prostate growth.

BPH, DHEA, AND PROSTATE CANCER

Men with BPH appear to be at increased risk for prostate cancer, although the extent of that risk is not known. We do know that over 80 percent of prostate cancers respond to androgen (male sex hormone) withdrawal, that is, the elimination of testosterone production by castration or the use of antitestosterone drugs such as estrogen.

DHEA *can be* converted to testosterone, but moderate doses raise testosterone very little. In fact, research shows that women convert more DHEA to testosterone than men do.

Is DHEA therefore risk-free in relation to BPH and prostate cancer? That remains to be seen, but consider that some men with BPH appear to *improve* when they receive moderate doses of DHEA, and clinicians monitoring male patients tell me that they see no increase in symptoms with low to moderate doses of DHEA.

Today a blood test can measure to some degree one's risk for prostate cancer. Levels of prostate specific antigen (PSA) reflect the level of abnormal cell proliferation in the gland, and neither clinicians nor researchers have found that DHEA supplements increase PSA. Still, some physicians recommend that male patients take saw palmetto supplements along with DHEA, and that may ultimately become common practice. In addition, most doctors will not prescribe DHEA for a man with symptoms of BPH or higher than normal levels of PSA. Clearly, this is something to discuss and monitor with your physician.

MENOPAUSE

No one knows why women experience menopause. Women certainly don't run out of eggs. A woman is born with approximately 600,000 immature eggs called *oocytes* nestled in her ovaries and will bring only about 400 to maturity in her lifetime.

Some believe that the ovaries stop producing estrogen and progesterone because they become "exhausted," but that makes no sense. A woman's pancreas works much harder than her ovaries do and can do so for 100 or more years. No, I favor the hard, cold evolutionary explanation: When a woman is past her prime strength and fitness years, DNA triggers the shutdown of her reproductive system.

Remember, we have Stone Age genes, and back in Paleolithic times a fifty-year-old woman was very old indeed, certainly not able to care for a newborn. And don't forget that menopause sets other decline systems in motion, such as accelerated bone loss, decreases in immunity, and increased risk for heart disease. Once again nature is saying, "Gee, it was nice having you on the planet. There's the door."

Will keeping DHEA levels at prime peak enable a woman to

postpone menopause? No one knows, but it makes perfect sense. In the limited clinical trials that have been completed with perimenopausal women (those in their late forties just starting to experience menopausal symptoms) DHEA administration resulted in restored menstrual regularity, heightened libido, and enhanced sexual enjoyment.

Experts attribute these benefits primarily to increased testosterone, but I suspect there is more to it than that. After all, giving a woman straight testosterone via injection, tablet, or transdermal patch does not appear to produce the same broad range of effects. Perhaps the best results will ultimately be derived from a combination of DHEA and estrogen, with the ratio of those substances changing with a woman's age.

THE BIG PICTURE

Freud, of course, was wrong. Libido is powerful and tremendously important for the experience of certain pleasures and the expression of what might be called the life force, but life is a balance and libido is not the be-all and end-all. There are times when other motivations and behaviors are more compelling and even more urgent. I spent six years in a yoga ashram as a monastic student because there were lessons I needed to learn that libido could not teach.

The good news is that we now have a choice and the tools to explore the further unfolding of libido into our forties, fifties, and beyond. The sex drive is not an on-off switch but a continuum of feelings, emotions, and behaviors that affect every aspect of our lives. Once again, there are those who will decry this development, claiming that humankind is too degenerate to handle this kind of choice, but I disagree. That's like saying you're glad your neighbor was robbed of her life savings because she would have spent the money unwisely.

As we go through life, we are slowly robbed of our energy and vitality. The DHEA Plan can help us regain that lost fortune, and I believe we should celebrate and make good use of those gifts. Remember that DHEA is a battery charger, not an aphrodisiac, which is true of the entire program. You will experience the benefits of youthfulness and vitality as your metabolic efficiency is enhanced and your cells start to produce more energy. It's not an artificial stimulation but *the fulfillment of your genetic potential for life.*

The image has been used many times, but it is perfectly accurate: Life is a symphony of experience. Freud heard only one note played over and over. If we fall into that mind-set, growing old will be terrifying with or without DHEA. The secret is to learn the important lessons along the way so that you can experience and contribute your best at every stage. Libido provides the bass notes, if you will, but a truly successful life requires the added harmony of wisdom, creativity, and compassion.

The tragedy has always been that we run out of time and/or energy just when we have gained that wisdom. Again, it's not just a matter of information but of motivation and capability. We know that exercise is important, but it becomes a struggle. The DHEA Plan makes exercise easier and more enjoyable at any age.

We want to have a positive outlook on life, but advancing age often brings chronic pain and depression. The following chapters will show you how to improve your mood naturally as well as prevent or eliminate a wide range of musculoskeletal pain by strengthening your joints, tendons, ligaments, and bones. The DHEA Plan can also sharpen your memory and cognition skills, and it holds great promise for reducing the degenerative changes that cripple our minds as we age.

THERE'S NO MAGIC BULLET

This is obviously not a "magic bullet" approach. You have to understand that no matter how attractive the "instant results" mentality may be, *it has never worked.* It's understandable. Life is complex, and so we naturally seek simple solutions: one pill that will do it all. But whenever researchers have tried to find the magic bullet, they have failed.

The most popular drugs in America right now are a group of antidepressants classified as selective serotonin reuptake inhibitors (SSRIs). More than 40 million prescriptions have been filled, mostly for women, yet a common side effect is sexual dysfunction: decreased libido, delayed orgasm, or inability to achieve orgasm.

Ultimately we as a society will see the big picture. It's not a single hormone or drug. It's not anything that you can buy, but what you do and how you live. An important new study found that sexual activity in older men and women is related more to physical activity and social and personality factors than to any hormone level. In other words, *don't rush out to buy DHEA*. Take a close look at your life. Are you an active participant, or have you fallen into the trap of being a spectator?

The entire DHEA Plan is geared toward getting you passionately and intensely involved with life. Today, if you are 50 years old, your chances of living to 100 are very good. But if you want those years to be active and vibrant, you have to take action now. Don't wait another twenty years, hoping for a miracle drug. It's time to wake up and start using the incredible resources we have available to change our lives for the better. Onward and upward!

BIBLIOGRAPHY

Anderson RA, Bancroft J, Wu FC. The effects of exogenous testosterone on sexuality and mood of normal men. *J Clin Endocrinol Metab* 1992; 75(6): 1503–7.

Bachmann GA. Influence of menopause on sexuality. *Int J Fertil Menopausal Stud* 1995; 40 (Suppl 1):16–22.

Brahler E, Unger U. Sexual activity in advanced age in the context of gender, family status and personality aspects—results of a representative survey. *Z Gerontol* 1994; 27(2):110–5.

Groeneveld FP, Bareman FP, Barentsen R, Dokter HJ, Drogendijk AC, Hoes AW. The climacteric and well-being. *J Psychosom Obstet Gynaecol* 1993; 14(2):127–43.

Rowland DL, Greenleaf WJ, Dorfman LJ, Davidson JM. Aging and sexual function in men. *Arch Sex Behav* 1993; 22(6):545–57.

Sadowsky M, Antonovsky H, Sobel R, Maoz B. Sexual activity and sex hormone levels in aging men. *Int Psychogeriatr* 1993; 5(2):181–6.

Sands R, Studd J. Exogenous androgens in postmenopausal women. *Am J Med* 1995; 98(1A):76S–9S.

Schiavi RC, Segraves RT. The biology of sexual function. *Psychiatr Clin North Am* 1995; 18(1):7–23.

Shen WW, Hsu JH. Female sexual side effects associated with selective serotonin reuptake inhibitors: A descriptive clinical study of 33 patients. *Int J Psychiatry Med* 1995; 25(3):239–48.

Swerdloff RS, Wang C. Androgen deficiency and aging in men. *West J Med* 1993; 159(5):579–85.

CHAPTER 3

Better Than Sex: Staying Alive

If your response to the title of this chapter is "What could be better than sex?" you're certainly young at heart but haven't given it enough thought. *Life itself* is better, or perhaps I should say more important, than sex. And the desire to stay alive is an equally strong motivating factor in human behavior.

In a way, the desire for longevity is a rebellion against the tyranny of our genes. As I explained in the introduction, nature cares little for the survival of an individual much past reproductive age. But *we* care and spend a great deal of time and resources trying to figure out how to prolong life.

As important as longevity is the *quality* of life. Few people would want to live 120 years if the last four decades were spent in chronic illness or pain. Thus, it excites me to know that we are on the threshold of major advances in quality-of-life research; once again DHEA is a major player.

This chapter explores some of the remarkable ways DHEA can help you survive, and *thrive*, longer than you ever thought possible. The DHEA-immunity connection is unfolding every week, and this chapter includes information that has never been assembled in print before.

BACKGROUND

Long before puberty DHEA is a key factor in *all* growth and development. Tissues throughout the body compete for available DHEA, and levels in the brain are six times those in any other tissue or organ. This has led some researchers to postulate that DHEA might have played a critical role in the evolution of higher mammals, as only humans and other primates are capable of producing large amounts of DHEA. Moreover, DHEA production appears to be directly proportional to the size of the brain, with humans producing the most.

Recent studies illustrate that DHEA is involved in DNA transcription, an essential process in cell repair and duplication. Thus, DHEA is not simply a growth stimulator but a growth *regulator*, a critical point to remember in looking at the relationship of DHEA and cancer. As you will see, DHEA has powerful anticancer activity, largely as a result of its ability to control abnormal cell proliferation.

The point is that scientists have been treating DHEA as a sex hormone simply because *that's the only place they have looked*. But in the last five years there has been a virtual explosion of DHEA research in physiology, biochemistry, general medicine, geriatrics, longevity, gynecology, immunology, and even neurochemistry. In fact, the specific enzymes necessary for the metabolism of DHEA are found in virtually every tissue of the human body.

It is therefore foolish to call DHEA a sex steroid. *It just may be, as one group of researchers claim, the "mother steroid" of all human life.*

STOPPING THE NUMBER-ONE KILLER

The term *cardiovascular disease* includes disorders of the heart and blood vessels. Atherosclerosis is the progressive blocking of an artery. If that artery leads to your heart, you have a heart attack. If it leads to your brain, you have a stroke. Either event can kill you or leave you paralyzed. Cardiovascular disease is the leading cause of death in the Western world, with more than 45 percent of all heart attacks occurring in people under sixty-five years of age.

What does that mean? Imagine that every day three jumbo jets crashed in the United States, each one packed with 450 passengers, and there was never a single survivor. That's the incredible toll cardiovascular disease takes in this country day after day after day.

Did you know that bypass surgery (in which a blocked coronary artery is replaced by a clean artery obtained from the thigh) is one of the biggest growth industries in the United States? Would it surprise you to learn that this procedure brings in more money to metropolitan hospitals than does any other type of care? In many cases bypass surgery accounts for *30 to 40 percent of a hospital's total income.*

The medical establishment refers to bypass surgery as "preventive care" even though studies show that bypass surgery does not extend overall life expectancy. (That's because the newly grafted artery usually starts clogging right away.)

Then there are the drugs used to lower blood pressure and cholesterol—another growth industry. These drugs are also called "preventive care" even though there are studies showing that individuals treated with them have *increased* overall mortality and even though an entire class of blood pressure medications has been shown to *increase the risk for heart attack.*

The jets keep crashing because nothing is being done to prevent it. I'm not a conspiracy nut, but this one is hard to ignore. There's an astronomical amount of money being made on treatments that provide very little benefit, *while the really effective therapies are largely ignored.*

FOR A HEALTHY HEART: VITAMIN E AND DHEA

You see, there are ways to prevent cardiovascular disease, but they are simple and inexpensive. In 1993 two remarkable studies were published in the *New England Journal of Medicine* showing that vitamin E can decrease heart disease risk by 26 to 46 percent. These conclusive studies followed more than a decade of similar research.

Now there's DHEA, which works in concert with vitamin E on a number of different levels. In 1986 a study published in the *New England Journal of Medicine* reported the following:

A 100 micrograms per deciliter increase in DHEA sulfate concentration corresponded with a 48 percent reduction in mortality due to cardiovascular disease and a 36 percent reduction in mortality for any reason. . . . those individuals with higher DHEA sulfate levels lived longer and had a much lower risk of heart disease.[1]

To grasp the extraordinary opportunity we now have to reduce needless suffering and death, you have to understand that heart disease is a multifaceted problem. It is not simply a cholesterol or blood pressure problem, although those factors play a role. You don't have clean arteries and then wake up one day with clogged arteries. Atherosclerosis proceeds along three well-understood stages, and *every one* of those stages is influenced by DHEA and/or vitamin E.

Stage One

Cholesterol is a fatty substance and, like all fats, can become rancid. A chemist would say it *oxidizes*. The oxidation of cholesterol in the bloodstream produces damaging free radicals that injure the lining of the artery. The body's response to this injury or lesion is now seen as the beginning of atherosclerosis. Later the injury site collects cellular debris, calcium, protein, and ultimately cholesterol to form the plaque that blocks blood flow. Vitamin E prevents the oxidation of cholesterol so that the initial injury does not occur. Now, *that's* prevention.

Stage Two

In the lining of an artery, abnormal cell production contributes to the atherosclerotic process. DHEA prevents this excessive cell proliferation, and this has been proved in tissue cultures, animals, and humans. In coronary patients, for example, those with arterial blockage greater than 50 percent were found to have lower DHEA levels than those without such extensive blockage. In fact, as blood levels of DHEA increased, there was a corresponding drop in the number of diseased blood vessels and the extent of coronary atherosclerosis.

To test this association further, researchers conducted a long-term study in patients who had undergone bypass surgery. Once again, blood levels of DHEA predicted the relative success of the surgery. In patients with low levels of DHEA, abnormal cell proliferation caused rapid degeneration of the new arteries.

Stage Three

As plaque accumulates in an artery, the result at first may be chest pain (angina) or ministrokes known as transient ischemic attacks (TIAs). Heart attacks and strokes are caused by a *complete* blockage that prevents oxygen from reaching the heart or brain, resulting in cell death. This blockage usually is caused by a clot that lodges in the narrowed artery, and these clots are commonly made up of blood cells called platelets.

Platelet aggregation is the rate at which platelets in the bloodstream clump. The natural adherence of platelets is critically important to normal clotting, but if they become too "sticky," they can form abnormal clots that greatly increase risk for heart attack and stroke. As is shown in the following chart, DHEA has been shown to decrease abnormal platelet aggregation. In one study, human volun-

THE DRAMATIC DECREASE IN PLATELET AGGREGATION IN MALE SUBJECTS AFTER THE ADDITION OF DHEA

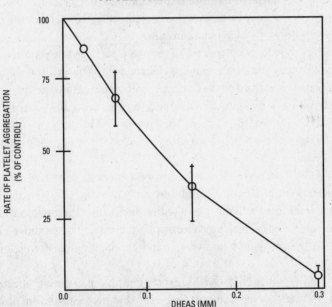

Reprinted by permission of The Annals of The New York Academy of Sciences from "Dehydroepiandrosterone Inhibits Human Platelet Aggregation In Vitro and In Vivo" by RL Jesse, et al., December 29, 1995, 774, pp. 281–290.

teers were given either DHEA or a placebo and then received a clottin-gagent. Those taking the DHEA experienced a remarkable decrease in platelet aggregation, even to the point of complete normalization, while none in the placebo group experienced such benefits.

In addition, recent research with human volunteers suggests another way in which DHEA may help prevent and even dissolve abnormal clots. After taking 50 mg of DHEA for only twelve days, a group of men showed an enhanced ability to dissolve fibrin, another structural component of blood clots.

ADDITIONAL FACTORS IN HEART DISEASE

Insulin Sensitivity

An important marker of aging is a gradual decrease in insulin sensitivity throughout the body. Remember that insulin is the hormone that "escorts" glucose and other fuels out of the bloodstream and into the tissues by binding to insulin receptors on the cell. When cells become less sensitive to insulin, this binding is impaired and the condition is termed *insulin resistance*. The cells still need fuel, but the body responds only by making more insulin.

Imagine you are desperate to receive a package but your doorbell is broken and you don't hear the deliveryman. You call the shipping company and scream at the manager, who sends out *two* deliverymen. Now you have two guys pressing your broken doorbell, but they also leave and you still don't have your package. This goes on until you finally notice that there are twenty deliverymen standing in your front yard.

When the body does this, you end up with elevated levels of insulin in your blood, a condition known as *hyperinsulinism*. This increases risk for a number of diseases, including atherosclerosis, diabetes, and obesity. Hyperinsulinism also contributes to cardiovascular disease by damaging blood vessels and accelerating the formation of plaque.

Studies show that DHEA exerts multiple preventive effects in this regard. A recent report suggests that hyperinsulinism lowers DHEA by accelerating *metabolic clearance*. In other words, excessive insulin somehow causes the body to use up DHEA at a faster rate, producing a "double whammy" of greater damage and less protection.

The authors of this study suggest that oral DHEA may break this vicious cycle and help prevent the major diseases associated with aging.

In fact, that appears to be true. A recent study with human volunteers measured insulin and glucose in response to a nightly dose of 100 mg of DHEA. After only thirty days insulin fell by 27 percent. This study also found that DHEA supplementation increased the levels of IGF-1. IGF-1 helps reduce the risk of heart attack by dilating the blood vessels and improving circulation. The exciting piece of that puzzle is the fact that IGF-1 levels also fall as we grow older. Once again, DHEA appears to be the master switch that turns on an entire cascade of antiaging benefits throughout the body.

Fat: On Your Thighs and in Your Blood

Overweight individuals have a fourfold greater risk for cardiovascular disease compared with those of normal weight. Much of this is due to the bad things that happen to fat (such as oxidation and the production of free radicals), but obesity also contributes to hyperinsulinism. In addition to the direct cardiovascular risks mentioned above, excessive insulin production causes wide swings in blood sugar and low exercise tolerance.

It is quite common for thin people to criticize those who are overweight for not exercising enough. However, it is important to recognize that human beings will not consistently do something that feels bad. Obesity makes exercise arduous and painful, while a high percentage of lean tissue makes exercise easy and enjoyable. We'll examine this important issue in detail in Chapter 7, but for now let's just look at the catch-22 obese individuals face.

Everyone tells them to exercise more, but excessive insulin secretion causes wide swings in blood sugar and profound fatigue. What's more, when obese individuals try to exercise, they become exhausted very quickly, and if they manage to complete an exercise routine, their joints and muscles ache the following day. Who would willingly repeat that torture on a regular basis?

The good news is that DHEA can help turn this situation around. In a landmark study designed to evaluate body fat, hormone, and cholesterol changes, normal-weight human volunteers were given a rather large daily dose of 1600 mg of DHEA for twenty-eight days.

There were no significant changes in the placebo group, but those taking DHEA showed a 31 percent mean reduction in the percentage of body fat, even though their overall weight did not decrease nearly as much. Clearly, DHEA supplementation produced a very significant increase in muscle mass. More muscle means greater metabolic efficiency, improved insulin sensitivity, greater exercise tolerance, and a decreased risk for cardiovascular disease.

Then there's fat in the bloodstream, which can be elevated even in very thin people. Obviously, when you have a high level of cholesterol in your blood, you have a greater chance of that cholesterol oxidizing no matter how much vitamin E you take. The specific form of cholesterol that produces this damage is the "bad" cholesterol known as low-density lipoprotein (LDL). The same study found that those taking DHEA enjoyed a 5 percent decrease in total cholesterol—very significant for a twenty-eight-day period. More important, this improvement was almost entirely due to a fall of 7.5 percent in the LDL component.

Gender

It is not clear whether gender is a factor in one's level of protection against heart disease. Unfortunately, most human studies relating to DHEA have been conducted with men. Studies with women have produced mixed results. One extensive evaluation of DHEA in postmenopausal women (the Rancho Bernardo study) found no significant protection against heart disease. Recently, however, another team of investigators found that decreases in insulin sensitivity could be nearly eliminated when a group of postmenopausal women were given 50 mg of DHEA per day. More research is needed to evaluate these inconsistencies and apparent gender differences before any conclusions can be reached.

DHEA AND YOUR HEART: A SUMMARY

Our understanding of cardiovascular disease as a complex disorder leads to the awareness that effective prevention can be achieved at numerous points, and recent research lends support to the idea that DHEA may be a pivotal factor. Men who survived heart attacks and symptom-free men with coronary artery disease were both found to have much lower DHEA levels than did healthy men of the same age.

The good news for men *and* women is that DHEA plays an important role in almost every preventive intervention, including reducing abnormal clot formation, increasing muscle mass, decreasing LDL cholesterol, and preventing the abnormal proliferation of arterial cells. Most important, these benefits appear to be obtainable from a moderate-dose DHEA supplement, and so the risk-reward ratio is extremely favorable.

ENHANCING GENERAL IMMUNITY

Imagine the complexity of the U.S. defense system: the training, administration, and functioning of the Army, Navy, Air Force, and Marines. Then add the intelligence-gathering agencies, rapid-response units, missile defense, Veterans Administration, research, and new weapons development. All that is child's play compared to your immune system.

You have somewhere in the neighborhood of 100 trillion cells in your body (roughly twenty thousand times the population of the earth), and your immune system will know if *one* of those cells does not belong there. Your immune system produces an array of weapons that would astound a brigadier general and constantly adjusts and modifies its response to fit the precise characteristics of an enemy. Even in victory your immune system never rests. Instead, it produces cells that remember every foe it has ever fought so that it will be more effective in repelling a future attack.

When it comes to enhancing immunity, this military analogy works well. For example, when a political candidate says she wants to strengthen defense, you can bet that her intention is to give the Defense Department *more money*. But we have seen in recent history that the Defense Department is capable of monumental waste. More money, in other words, does not guarantee better defense. Defense is more complicated than that.

Similarly, we must resist the temptation to see the immune system as something we can easily tweak. When suffering with an illness, we all like to think that we can go to the health store and buy pills that will "boost" immunity, but it doesn't work that way. While it is safe to say that correcting poor nutrient levels will enhance immunity, most of the "immune" products in health stores are unproven and some are dangerous. Again, this is because immunity is extraordinarily complex. You cannot simply throw vitamins at it and expect to achieve true enhancement. In some cases augmenting one aspect of immunity will have negative effects on another "branch" of the defense system.

THE IMMUNE "BALANCE"

The point is that immune enhancement is not simply immune stimulation. That's because immunity is a *balance*, not an on-off switch. Over the years a number of pharmaceutical agents have purported to boost immunity, such as the interleukins, but all have proved to have limited value and significant risk. Cranking up the immune system, for example, can make your allergies worse or accelerate autoimmune disorders such as rheumatoid arthritis, lupus, and multiple sclerosis.

What makes DHEA so attractive is that it appears to restore immune *balance*. Immunologists use the term *up-regulating* to describe this enhancement and point excitedly to research showing that the overall immune profile of an old mouse can be restored to that of a young mouse simply by feeding the mouse DHEA. That's a world of difference compared with an agent that simply causes the immune system to go into hyperdrive. But there's also a world of difference between mice and people. Let's look at some important new studies that are applicable to humans.

Monocyte Activation

Immune cells called *monocytes* play a pivotal role in the body's response to a wide variety of organisms, including viruses and, most important, cancer cells. They attack tumor cells directly and also stimulate the production of *other* potent anticancer biochemicals such as interferon, tumor necrosis factor (TNF), and reactive oxygen (free radicals).

Keep in mind that none of these immune weapons can be administered *directly* to the human body without significant risk, but a substance that enhances monocyte activity or increases monocyte production can provide tremendous benefits. That substance is DHEA. Recent research has shown that DHEA administration increases monocyte production and that these cells are more active in defending the body. In fact, scientists mapping the submicroscopic details of monocyte cells recently discovered a specific binding site for DHEA, confirming a direct relationship between DHEA and immune competence.

B Cells

When elderly human volunteers were given 50 mg of DHEA over a six-month period, there was a "functional activation" of B cells, meaning that those cells reacted more swiftly and powerfully to defend the body against a large number of disease-causing organisms.

T Cells

T cells, or T lymphocytes, play an important role in your immune system. Unlike B cells, which use antibody "missiles" to seek and destroy specific targets, the T cell is more like a heavily armed foot soldier ready for just about any enemy. Most people have heard of T cells because they are the immune cells destroyed by the AIDS virus. But T cells are involved in just about *every* immune response from simple infection to life-threatening disease.

Almost a decade ago scientists noted improvements in T-cell numbers and activity in AIDS patients who were given supplemental DHEA. A recent study in the *Journal of Clinical Endocrinology and Metabolism* offers a tentative explanation. Scientists have found binding sites specific for the DHEA molecule on human T cells, and they have concluded that these immune cells may be regulated by DHEA. In other words, when T cells are mobilized to fight infection or disease, DHEA is a critical factor in determining the strength of the defensive effort.

We now know at least one specific way in which DHEA boosts T-cell function. A landmark study published in the *Annals of the New York Academy of Sciences* found that supplementing elderly individuals with DHEA increased T-cell production of two powerful immune weapons known as interleukin-2 and gamma-interferon. Clearly, this indicates that the progressive weakening of immunity that accompanies aging may be modified significantly and perhaps reversed. If so, it will represent one of the most important advances in the field of preventive medicine in the twentieth century.

The Thymus

The name *T cell* comes from the fact that these lymphocytes, for some unknown reason, migrate to the thymus gland soon after they are formed. There they are transformed from normal, everyday lymphocytes into powerful, highly effective soldiers. Think of the thymus as a special forces training academy for motivated immune cells.

However, the thymus tends to shrink as we age, and so therefore does immune competence. One can slow the shrinking of the thymus through optimum nutrition, regular exercise, and not smoking, but recent studies suggest that more can be done. It turns out that the maintenance of thymic mass depends on growth hormone (GH) secreted by the pituitary. GH levels start dropping soon after puberty, signaling the body to stop growing. By age fifty GH production in most individuals is too low to measure, and the thymus is well on its way to becoming a shriveled shadow of its former self.

Even though growth is no longer needed, the body must still be involved in continual repair and maintenance. To accomplish this, the liver and other tissues produce IGF-1. IGF-1 has been shown to stimulate thymus growth, but we're not out of the woods yet, because the production of IGF-1 also declines with age. Enter DHEA. DHEA is a powerful stimulant of IGF-1 production, and research suggests that it can prevent and in some cases reverse the atrophy and shrinking of the thymus.

There's more. Certain hormones known as *glucocorticoids* actively suppress thymus function and accelerate the involution or shrinking of that gland. Glucocorticoids such as cortisol are produced by the adrenals in response to stress. Others, such as prednisone and dexamethasone, are used in medicine. In animal experiments scientists have been able to block about 50 percent of glucocorticoid-induced immune suppression by administering DHEA. This suggests that some of the many immune benefits associated with DHEA may be due to its opposing or buffering effect on glucocorticoids.

Some researchers believe that this buffering of glucocorticoids will turn out to be the main benefit of DHEA because continuing research is revealing more and more ways in which stress hormones suppress immunity. In addition to accelerating the demise of the thymus, glucocorticoids interfere with the immune system's ability to turn on specific genes to mount an effective immune response. DHEA also appears to neutralize that effect. In a recent experiment mice were exposed to an intestinal bacteria and then were given either prednisone or DHEA. The prednisone group had a 25 percent survival rate, while 72 percent of the DHEA group survived.

NK Cells

Remember the movie *Dirty Harry?* It opens with Clint Eastwood sitting at a lunch counter across the street from a bank. To anyone else the scene looks perfectly normal, but Clint senses that something's amiss. He tells the waiter to call the police and then saunters over to the bank, gun drawn, just as the robbers burst out the front door.

This is the story of cancer and your immune system. Cancer cells have a unique ability to cloak their nefarious activity. After they reach a certain number, they produce a protein coating that literally hides the rapid growth of malignant cells from the immune system. But then there are Dirty Harry cells known as natural killer (NK) cells. You're beginning to get the picture.

NK cells have two things that other immune cells don't have. One is that, just like Harry, they don't need to be called; they just *know* when something's wrong. Second, just like Harry, they have weapons the normal police don't have. A colony of cancer cells may look perfectly normal to an ordinary leukocyte, but when an NK cell passes by, it senses that something's not right. Then, just like Harry, the cell utilizes a high-powered weapon to blow a hole in the colony's protein coat. At that point the police (other immune cells) arrive and say: "Holy cow, there's cancer in there!"and all hell breaks loose.

NK cells are also very active against viruses. These are cells you want to have around, and knowing their value, researchers have worked hard to find ways to increase their numbers and activity. They met with little success until 1993, when a group led by Peter Casson at the University of Tennessee found that DHEA produced "dramatic" increases in NK cell strength in human volunteers. Importantly, the subjects were postmenopausal women, and the amount of

DHEA that produced these remarkable results was a *physiologic* dose, that is, a dose approximating DHEA levels in a healthy young person. Dr. Samuel Yen and his colleagues at the University of California in San Diego documented similar benefits in elderly men with a nightly DHEA dose of 50 mg.

The activation of NK cells was precisely the model everyone had been looking for, because it provides a rationale for the anticancer benefits many researchers had observed earlier. In fact, Casson and his colleagues argue that the age-related decrease in DHEA production in both men and women might well be termed "adrenopause," helping explain why cancer incidence increases dramatically as we grow older.

DHEA AND CANCER

Population studies show that low levels of DHEA are associated with cancer of the stomach, breast, prostate, and bladder. This fact may be meaningless. After all, just because two events are associated does not mean that one causes the other. If, however, there is a cause-and-effect relationship, we may be looking at an important way to reduce the risk of cancer. Let's see if we can make that determination.

Step One: How Reliable Is the Association?

The association of low DHEA and cancer has been reported by more than a dozen authors. As early as 1962, investigators in Great Britain reported low DHEA in women who developed breast cancer, and the association was apparent as long as nine years before the diagnosis. Another long-term study found low DHEA levels in women who later developed ovarian cancer. Still, at least one contrary study was recently published by the *Journal of the American Medical Association* in which women with ovarian cancer were found to have *higher* levels of DHEA than did age-matched controls.

Step Two: Does the Association Work Both Ways?

People with low levels of DHEA appear to have greater risk for developing certain cancers, but is it also true that a high level of DHEA confers protection? To answer this, researchers first used test-tube models of cancer growth and found DHEA to have remarkable anticancer activity.

Step Three: Does the Administration of DHEA Lower Cancer Incidence in Animals?

Once again the answer is yes. Researchers have reliable ways to induce cancer in a variety of animals, and some rat strains are genetically "programmed" to get cancer. When these experimental and cancer-prone animals are fed DHEA, the incidence of cancer is reduced significantly and in some cases eliminated completely.

Step Four: How Can We Evaluate Confounding or Contrary Data?

This is where the cancer-DHEA connection becomes unclear. Besides the conflicting results relating to ovarian cancer, clinicians and researchers disagree about the risk for other hormone-responsive tumors, such as those of the prostate and breast. One group, for example, found a decreased risk for breast cancer (in laboratory cell cultures) as a result of DHEA's ability to block estrogen receptors. Others, however, are concerned about a possible breast cancer–*promoting* effect from the conversion of DHEA to testosterone and estradiol (both risk factors for breast cancer when elevated). Huge doses of DHEA have caused liver cancer in mice, and the standard therapy for advanced prostate cancer is drug therapy to reduce the levels of *all* androgens, including DHEA.

SUMMARY: DHEA'S ANTICANCER BENEFITS

The preponderance of evidence supports a protective role of DHEA in many types of cancer. Anticancer activity has been demonstrated in animal models of skin, lung, colon, breast, prostate, and lymphatic cancer. In most cases the results have been dramatic. In a study published recently in the journal *Cancer Research* investigators exposed mice to a treatment that would normally induce breast cancer. Indeed, more than 70 percent of the control group developed breast cancer. In the group given DHEA *not one animal* developed the disease.

There are a number of solid explanations of *how* DHEA exerts this anticancer activity. Numerous investigators have found that DHEA inhibits the enzyme glucose-6-phosphate dehydrogenase (G6PDH), which is required for cancer growth. This inhibition is so effective that you can inject it, apply it topically, or put it in the animal's food; however you get DHEA into an animal, it will significantly reduce the incidence of cancer. DHEA also possesses *antioxidant* activity, which can help limit cancer in the initial stages.

However, test tube studies and animal experiments have taken us as far as we can go. We desperately need studies in which groups of men and women are given either DHEA or a look-alike placebo and followed for ten or fifteen years. Research also needs to evaluate the benefits of techniques that can optimize the body's own DHEA production. Only then will we know for certain exactly what anticancer benefits one can expect from DHEA.

With overall cancer incidence on the rise, you might expect that these studies would be under way by now. Unfortunately, that is not the case. Worse, the necessary studies may *never* happen, because DHEA is an unpatentable "orphan drug" and no pharmaceutical company will fund the research. Such is the state of affairs when profit is the driving force behind health research.

Nevertheless, many individuals and doctors are not waiting for rock-solid proof. I know physicians who are using DHEA as part of an overall treatment program for cancer. Others have found it beneficial to their patients but hesitate to use it in cases of breast, ovarian, or prostate cancer. One thing is certain: Professional guidance is *absolutely necessary* if you have cancer or if you're at high risk.

CANCER, CHOLESTEROL, AND DHEA: AN INTRIGUING HYPOTHESIS

For over a decade researchers have puzzled over the fact that abnormally low cholesterol levels are associated with certain types of cancer. Once again, the questions arise: Is low cholesterol a risk factor for cancer? Does cancer cause blood cholesterol levels to drop? I believe that DHEA provides the solution to this mystery.

GIVEN: All steroid hormones, including DHEA, are derived from cholesterol. In the case of DHEA the intermediate hormone is pregnenolone. So chemically it looks like this:

Cholesterol→(is metabolized to) pregnenolone→(which is metabolized to) DHEA.

GIVEN: Cancer cells are the most rapidly growing cells in the human body. Chemotherapeutic drugs are agents that kill rapidly proliferating cells.

GIVEN: DHEA has profound antiproliferative activity. That is, it works to control abnormal cell growth.

GIVEN: Decreases in blood cholesterol levels are observed primarily in the early or preclinical stages of cancer.

PROPOSED: When cancer is growing, cholesterol is needed to form the cell membranes of the rapidly proliferating cells. This drain on available cholesterol lowers blood levels and also decreases the conversion of cholesterol to DHEA.

PROPOSED: This is the triple whammy of cancer.

1. Cancer cell proliferation depletes cholesterol, which is the precursor to DHEA, the very substance that would limit cancer growth. DHEA is selectively lowered because cortisol (an adrenal stress hormone) is preferentially produced in response to the metabolic stress.

2. Low levels of DHEA are associated with impaired NK cell activity. Remember that NK cells are the body's primary anticancer weapon.

3. As cancer growth continues unchecked, the levels of stress hormones such as cortisol increase further, producing a downward spiral of immune suppression and decreasing DHEA (see Chapter 4).

A RATIONAL APPROACH

When DHEA is kept at prime peak levels, any fluctuation in the availability of cholesterol will not affect the body's anticancer capabilities. Inhibition of G6PDH will be maintained, as will NK cell activity. Such a strategy can be employed without resorting to high doses of DHEA, but it involves consulting a physician who is willing to monitor levels of DHEA and the other parameters outlined in Chapter 11.

Remember that low DHEA is strongly associated with cancer and even predictive of ultimate death from cancer. At the very least, it makes sense to do everything you can to maintain optimum production of DHEA by your body (see Chapter 4).

AIDS

When the human immunodeficiency virus (HIV) infects people, it sets about to weaken their immune systems, specifically targeting a group of T cells known as helper/inducer cells. The medical term for this group is CD4 cells. The progression to AIDS is accompanied by a continual decline in CD4 populations to the point where the body is no longer able to defend itself from bacterial, viral, fungal, or parasitic invaders. Infections that a healthy immune system would be able to conquer become life-threatening or fatal to a person with AIDS.

However, it is intriguing to note that if you put the HIV virus in a test tube with CD4 cells, the virus does not attack the immune cells. Therefore, there must be an intermediate step in the destruction of these important cells.

It has been known for some time that decreased production of adrenal steroids such as DHEA is associated with impaired immunity. When DHEA levels were measured in a group of HIV-positive men, not only was DHEA lower in the HIV-positive men compared to controls, but this was correlated in a perfect linear relationship with CD4 counts. As DHEA levels rose, so did the CD4 count.

While this gives us no conclusive picture, it strongly supports other evidence that DHEA is critical for optimal immune function and that decreased production contributes to the advancement of disease. What you and I are wondering at this moment is whether supplemental DHEA will be effective in the treatment of AIDS. That remains to be seen. But let's look at another intriguing piece of the puzzle.

THE DHEA-CORTISOL RELATIONSHIP

In the study just referred to, DHEA levels were inversely related to cortisol, meaning that as cortisol increased, DHEA decreased. This has been noted by numerous investigators, suggesting once again that under chronic stress the adrenals shift activity from DHEA to cortisol. Some experts believe that this may be the single most important mechanism in explaining the well-known stress-induced impairment of immunity. But how would that affect the progression of AIDS?

Researchers have found that DHEA is a "modest inhibitor" of HIV replication, meaning that it doesn't stop the virus from duplicating but slows down the process. Even more important is the fact that cortisol, the body's primary glucocorticoid hormone, accelerates HIV replication. There appears to be a "tug-of-war" in the bodies of HIV-positive individuals between cortisol and DHEA. To the degree that cortisol wins, the disease progresses. In support of this hypothesis, a report was recently published entitled "HIV and the Cortisol Connection: A Feasible Concept of the Process of AIDS."

This is not far-fetched. It is well known that glucocorticoids suppress immune function, including T cells. And it is not merely the fact that someone with AIDS would naturally be under a great deal of stress. Evidence suggests that the HIV virus *causes* the hyperactive secretion of cortisol. This may be the intermediate step everyone has been looking for, and it would certainly imply that DHEA supplementation may be extremely helpful in managing the disease.

Finally, there is the thymus itself, the factory where T cells are made. As was mentioned above, DHEA's stimulation of IGF-1 can enhance thymus growth and repair, thus restoring the production of T cells and building immune competence.

VACCINE AMPLIFICATION

Disease-causing organisms are collectively referred to as *pathogens*. When one invades the body, the immune system goes into attack mode and produces memory cells called *antibodies* to catalogue all the characteristics of that particular enemy. Thus, any subsequent exposure to the pathogen will be met with a more swift and effective defense.

Vaccines contain weak or dead strains of a pathogen that provide the immune system with just enough information to create antibodies. This "education" confers resistance to or immunity against future exposures to that particular pathogen, whether it be a bacteria, a virus, or another invader.

As we grow older, however, the immune system changes. The defense against old enemies (the recall response) may remain intact, but the development of new antibodies (the primary immune response) declines dramatically. In fact, a recent study published by the New York Academy of Sciences states, "The marked reduction in the ability to stimulate primary immune responses in the elderly has become the hallmark of immunosenescence in humans."

Is this a serious problem? Consider that even today influenza sends tens of thousands of people to the hospital every year. And 80 to 90 percent of influenza-associated deaths occur in people over age sixty-four. An agent that would improve the effectiveness of this one vaccine would save lives and reduce suffering.

Encouraged by the extraordinary success of animal studies, researchers recently conducted an experiment with elderly human volunteers to see if adding DHEA to a vaccine could improve antibody production. Administration of 50 mg of DHEA on the vaccine day and another 50 mg the following day produced marked improvement over a control group that was given a look-alike placebo. The difference, in fact, was so significant that the researchers concluded:

> The effectiveness of DHEA augmentation in reducing some of the more profound changes in immune function in the aged has led us to conclude that some of the previously described age-related alterations in immunity may be fully reversible.[2]

DIABETES

Diabetes is a condition in which a person is unable to control the level of sugar (glucose) in the blood. It's one of the major causes of death in the United States and results from a dysfunction in insulin metabolism, not simply, as many people think, from an insulin deficiency.

Type I diabetes is usually related to insufficient insulin production, but type II diabetes (adult-onset diabetes) is far more common and stems more from a decreased sensitivity of the body's cells to the insulin molecule. This is termed *insulin resistance*, and whether it leads to diabetes or not, most of us suffer from some degree of insulin resistance as we age.

As you will see, this has profound effects (none of them good) on a number of tissues, organs, and systems in the body. Exercise improves insulin sensitivity, and a sedentary lifestyle makes it worse. Weight gain, which is common as we grow older, also contributes directly to insulin resistance, as do stress and a high-sugar diet.

More than a decade ago researchers found that the administration of DHEA to diabetic mice could restore insulin sensitivity and literally "cure" the condition. For some reason, it took nine years for experiments to be conducted with humans, and definitive work has *still* not been done. If that surprises you, look into the diabetic drug market and see how many pharmaceuticals came out in the same period.

But research is progressing. In 1993 a single case report was published showing that DHEA could significantly improve insulin metabolism in a diabetic human. In 1995 two studies were conducted in nondiabetic postmenopausal women. In both cases supplementation with 50 mg of DHEA per day produced significant improvements in insulin sensitivity.

What remains to be done—actually, what researchers are begging to do if they can get the funds—is to give DHEA to a large number of adult-onset diabetic patients (male and female) and evaluate the results. In the meantime, there are plenty of physicians who are impressed enough with the animal research and secure enough about safety to work with their diabetic patients using DHEA.

I must point out that it is not only a matter of using DHEA supplements. Stress management, as you will see in Chapter 4, can have profound effects on DHEA and cortisol levels, and this (along with obesity and exercise) is at the very core of type II diabetes. Stress increases the production of cortisol, which stimulates the liver to release glucose into the bloodstream. Continual or chronic stress tends to keep blood sugar and insulin levels high. Managing stress is therefore the critical first step, to be followed by DHEA supplements if you do not achieve prime peak levels of DHEA with stress management alone.

ASTHMA

Asthma is another disorder whose incidence is increasing in America. The number of cases is increasing, but what is alarming to public health experts is that *mortality* is also increasing. The death rate from asthma has doubled in the last fifteen years.

There are a number of theories about why this is happening. Pollution levels are increasing, more people have pets, and stress levels are on the rise. All these are common asthma "triggers," but there are also indications that the drugs commonly used during an asthma "attack" may increase the severity of the disease over time.

The DHEA connection is compelling because it ties into numerous aspects of asthma. First of all, asthma is often treated with glucocorticoid medications, which we know tend to reduce DHEA. Studies show that asthma patients who use these drugs have low DHEA levels.

But even without taking glucocorticoid drugs, asthmatic patients have been found to have lower DHEA levels than do matched controls. This is intriguing, but it does not prove that taking DHEA will ameliorate asthma. Still, many clinicians are giving it a try, and conclusive research will be conducted before long. One thing is for certain, however: Stress management can increase your body's production of DHEA. Stress management can also decrease the incidence and severity of asthma. This seems like a good place to start.

CHRONIC FATIGUE

As far as I know, there is no published research on the use of DHEA for chronic fatigue, but many of the physicians I speak with are using it successfully. Here is the rationale. Chronic fatigue, also known as chronic fatigue immune dysfunction syndrome (CFIDS), is a multifaceted disorder involving abnormalities in the immune, hormone, bioenergetic, and nervous systems. DHEA is a powerful and prolific hormone that has regulating and restoring effects in all those areas.

The downward spiral of CFIDS is frightening, and I am not saying that DHEA is the panacea. But remission of symptoms appears to come from a treatment plan that affects as many points as possible on that spiral. Patients, for example, who need glucocorticoid drugs would normally suffer in the long term because of the drugs' immune-suppression side effects. DHEA can block those side effects.

CFIDS patients find exercise almost impossible, and so they rapidly lose fitness and muscle mass—the very things that could help them improve. DHEA raises levels of IGF-1, a powerful muscle-building biochemical that maximizes the metabolic benefits of even modest amounts of exercise. DHEA helps restore immune balance and manage stress and has far-reaching effects on mind, mood, and behavior. Together with the bioenergetics nutrients discussed in Chapter 6, it can, I believe, play an important role in the overall treatment of CFIDS.

LUPUS: SYSTEMIC LUPUS ERYTHEMATOSUS

Lupus is a disorder in which the immune system attacks the body's connective tissue as a result of the production of autoantibodies (antibodies targeting normal healthy tissue). Symptoms include profound fatigue, swollen glands, headaches, and the inflammation and swelling of joints. Skin rashes are also common. Hair loss, kidney damage, and neurological problems may ultimately appear.

Interestingly, 90 percent of lupus patients are women, suggesting a possible hormonal factor, but the cause has not been found. All that can be determined is that the immune system is "out of whack." In addition to the production of autoantibodies, levels of interleukin-2 (IL-2) are markedly reduced. Why that happens and what can be done to correct or prevent these defects remain to be seen.

Once again there is an intriguing DHEA connection. Actually, it's more than intriguing—it's extremely promising. First, lupus patients uniformly have low levels of DHEA compared with matched controls. Second, in the animal model of lupus researchers have found that oral administration of DHEA prevents the formation of autoantibodies and prolongs survival. Encouraged by this successful work, another group studied the effects of a 200 mg daily dose of DHEA in human lupus patients. They reported significant improvements in symptoms, a reduction of steroid drug requirements, and restored IL-2 production.

Still, even with this remarkable scientific foundation spanning more than a decade, research on DHEA and lupus (and other auto-immune disorders, such as rheumatoid arthritis) is proceeding at a snail's pace. If you would like to help change that, the address of the National Institutes of Health and the major lupus foundations are listed in Appendix B. Input from the public does count when research dollars are being apportioned.

INDIRECT IMMUNE SUPPORT

So far the discussion of immunity has been very direct. There is a defect, you do something to fix the defect, and you restore health. But in reality, as I pointed out at the beginning of this chapter, immunity is rarely so simple. There are a host of indirect influences that can favorably or unfavorably affect immune strength and balance. But even here DHEA can play a role.

Look at the immune-stimulating effects of exercise. For decades experts wondered why people who exercise regularly experience fewer illnesses compared with their sedentary friends. It turns out that a major factor is the transient (limited) fever they produce on a daily basis when they exercise. We've come to view fever as a bad thing. We rush to the medicine chest to lower a fever, when in fact the body produced that fever to crank up the immune response.

People who exercise to the point of raising their core body temperature give themselves a "fever" that may last only a few minutes, but it's enough to enhance overall immunity. The next time you break a sweat riding your bicycle or mowing the lawn, think about the millions of immune cells being activated by the effort.

Call me psychic, but I'll bet that some of you right now are wondering if you can just sit in a sauna or hot tub and get the same bene-fits. The answer is no. Saunas and hot tubs only raise the temperature of the *surface* of your body, and while they may provide some detoxi-fying benefits from profuse sweating, they will not stimulate immunity. You have to exercise for that.

And here's the DHEA connection. To exercise hard enough or long enough to produce the increased core body temperature, you need muscles. DHEA is a powerful muscle builder; I'm talking not about "Arnold" muscles but about muscle tone and strength, the things that get harder to maintain as we get older.

If you've fallen into the sedentary trap or lost your motivation because exercise is too difficult or too painful, tap into the metabolic boost DHEA and bioenergetics can provide (see Chapter 6). You'll be doing your heart, brain, and immune system a big favor.

CONCLUSION

As baby boomers age, more and more research is being conducted in gerontology, especially related to the decline in immune function. I have watched as research teams identified decreased activity of T cells, B cells, antibody production, and antitumor activity. But this is not simply a *lowering* of the immune response. Investigators have also found that immune *dysfunction* increases as we age. Autoimmune diseases increase, and the intricate relationship of the immune cells becomes unbalanced.

Each research team tries to identify the cause of this decline or dysfunction, but they all limit the search to the particular cell that they are studying, missing the larger picture. I believe that DHEA is the larger, unifying picture, and I suggest that it relates to my original scenario of DHEA as an aging clock.

In youth, DHEA floods every tissue in the human body, most notably the brain, the reproductive, and immune systems. When we pass the reproductive age, our bodies gradually decrease the production of DHEA. It's nature's way of giving us a few more decades so that we can care for the offspring we have created. In the advanced years, however, DHEA levels drop below an invisible threshold that triggers a widespread failure of immunity. What better way to remove an aging organism to make room for a younger, stronger one?

That's the "why," but we also need to know the "how" if we want to change that scenario. A group of researchers at the University of Utah School of Medicine believes it has found the secret. It has to do with the regulation of a group of immune proteins known as cytokines.

Cytokines are an integral part of the highly structured and coordinated workings of the immune system. Most important, they play a vital role in the way the immune system interacts with other systems and tissues. Their action is usually very local, sometimes affecting only a handful of cells, and extremely time-specific. A biochemist would call them "transient intercellular signaling molecules," and as such, they provide information to virtually every tissue and organ system in the body.

As was mentioned in the discussion of lupus, the immune system often becomes dysfunctional as we age. The production of cytokines such as interleukin-2 is decreased, while others are produced in excess. Weakening of bones, chronic inflammation, and increased production of autoantibodies (antibodies that target the body's own cells) are just a few of the effects of this imbalance. These effects in turn produce osteoporosis, an impaired immune response, certain types of cancer, and autoimmune disorders such as lupus, rheumatoid arthritis, and multiple sclerosis.

An agent that could restore cytokine balance would have far-reaching effects on aging and longevity. According to Dr. Nina Spencer and her colleagues, that agent is DHEA. Their research shows conclusively that at least in aged animals, DHEA administration can correct cytokine imbalance and restore normal immune competence. They conclude:

> The effects of DHEA . . . in aging might represent the elusive linchpin needed to provide investigators with a cohesive explanation for the diverse biologic activities of this steroid.[3]

If the results of animal studies continue to be documented in humans, we can expect that maintaining prime peak levels of DHEA may increase longevity from 25 to 50 percent. What excites me is that this increase in longevity to the 120-year mark and beyond could be accompanied by an increase in immune strength so that those extra years will be filled with health instead of pain and suffering.

There is one more piece of the immune and aging puzzle that remains to be explored. Once again it involves DHEA directly, and once again it is cutting-edge material that can change your life forever. It's the body-mind connection, what scientists are now referring to as *psychoneuroimmunology*. After reading this chapter, how do you feel about stress management? Would you like to know how you can double your DHEA level and decrease your stress level at the same time? Then turn to the next chapter.

BIBLIOGRAPHY

Barret-Connor E, Goodman-Gruen D. Dehydroepiandrosterone sulfate does not predict cardiovascular death in postmenopausal women: The Rancho Bernardo Study. *Circulation* 1995; 91(6):1757–60.

Barret-Conner E, Knaw KT, Yen SSC. A prospective study of dehydroepiandrosterone sulfate, mortality and cardiovascular disease. *N Engl J Med* 1986; 315:1519–24.

Bates GW Jr., Egerman RS, Umstot ES, Buster JE, Casson PR. Dehydroepiandrosterone attenuates study-induced declines in insulin sensitivity in postmenopausal women. *Ann NY Acad Sci* 1995; 774:291–3.

Beer NA, Jakubowicz DJ, Matt DW, Beer RM, Nestler JE. Dehydroepiandrosterone reduces plasma plasminogen activator inhibitor type 1 and tissue plasminogen activator antigen in men. *Am J Med Sci* 1996; 311(5):205–10.

Berrino F, Muti P, Micheli A, Bolelli G, Krogh V, Sciajno R, Pisani P, Panico S, Secreto G. Serum sex hormone levels after menopause and subsequent breast cancer. *JNCI* 1996; 88(5):291–6.

Buffington CK, Pourmotabbed G, Kitabachi AE. Case report: Amelioration of insulin resistance in diabetes with dehydroepiandrosterone. *Am J Med Sci* 1993; 306:320–4.

Bulbrook RD, Hayward JL, Spicer CC. Abnormal excretion of urinary steroids by women with early breast cancer. *Lancet* 1962; 2:1238–40.

Bulbrook RD, Hayward JL, Spicer CC. Relation between urinary androgen and corticoid excretion and subsequent breast cancer. *Lancet* 1971; 2:395–8.

Casson PR, Anderson RN, Herrod HG, et al. Oral dehydroepiandrosterone in physiologic doses modulates immune function in postmenopausal women. *Am J Obstet Gynecol* 1993; 169:1536–9.

Casson PR, Faquin L, Stentz F, et al. Replacement of DHEA enhances T-lymphocyte insulin binding in postmenopausal women. *Fertil Steril* 1995; 63(5):1027–31.

Cleary MP, Zabel T, Sartin JL. Effects of short-term dehydroepiandrosterone treatment on serum and pancreatic insulin in Zucker rats. *J Nutr* 1988; 118:382–7.

Coleman DL, Leiter EH, Applezweig N. Therapeutic effects of dehydroepiandrosterone metabolites in diabetic mice. *Endocrinology* 1984; 115:239–43.

Corley PA. HIV and the cortisol connection: A feasible concept of the process of AIDS. *Med Hypoth* 1995; 44(6):483–9.

Cuzick J, Bulstrode J, Stratton I, Thomas B, Bulbrook R, Hayward J. A prospective study of urinary androgen levels and ovarian cancer. *Int J Cancer* 1983; 32:723–6.

Danenberg HD, Ben-Yehuda A, Zakay-Rones Z, Friedman G. Dehydroepiandrosterone (DHEA) treatment reverses the impaired immune response of old mice to influenza vaccination and protects from influenza infection. *Vaccine* 1995; 13(15):1445–8.

Gianotti L, Alexander JW, Fukushima R, Pyles T. Steroid therapy can modulate gut barrier function, host defense, and survival in thermally injured mice. *J Surg Res* 1996; 62(1):53–8.

Gordon GB, Shantz LM, Talalay P. Modulation of growth, differentiation and carcinogenesis by dehydroepiandrosterone. *Adv Enzyme Regul* 1987; 26:355–82.

Helzlsouer K, Alberg A, Gordon G, Longcope C. Serum gonadotropins and steroid hormones and the development of ovarian cancer. *JAMA* 1995; 274:1926–30.

Henderson E, Yang JY, Schwartz A. Dehydroepiandrosterone (DHEA) and synthetic DHEA analogs are modest inhibitors of HIV-1 IIIB replication. *AIDS Res Hum Retroviruses* 1992; 8:625–31.

Herrington DM. Dehydroepiandrosterone and coronary atherosclerosis. *Ann NY Acad Sci* 1995; 774:271–80.

Hursting SD, Perkins SN, Haines DC, Ward JM, Phang JM. Chemoprevention of spontaneous tumorigenesis in p53-knockout mice. *Cancer Res* 1995; 55(18):3949–53.

Jakubowicz DJ, Beer N, Rengifo R. Effect of dehydroepiandrosterone on cyclic-guanosine monophosphate in men of advancing age. *Ann NY Acad Sci* 1995; 774:312–15.

Janero DR, Burghardt B. Oxidative injury to myocardial membrane: Direct modulation by endogenous alpha-tocopherol. *J Mole Cell Cardiol* 1989; 21(11):1111–24.

Jesse RL, Loesser K, Eich DM, Qian YZ, Hess ML, Nestler JE. Dehydroepiandrosterone inhibits human platelet aggregation in vitro and in vivo. *Ann NY Acad Sci* 1995; 774:281–90.

Laudat A, Blum L, Guechot J, Picard O, Cabane J, Imbert JC, Giboudeau J. Changes in systematic gonadal and adrenal steroids in asymptomatic human immunodeficiency virus-infected men: Relationship with the CD4 cell counts. *Eur J Endocrinol* 1995; 133(4):418–24.

Li S, Yan X, Belanger A, Labrie F. Prevention by dehydroepiandrosterone of the development of mammary carcinoma induced by 7,12-dimethylbenz(a)anthracene (DMBA) in the rat. *Breast Cancer Res Treat* 1993; 29:203–17.

Lucas JA, Ansar AS, Casey L, Mac Donald PC. Prevention of autoantibody formation and prolonged survival in New Zealand Black/New Zealand White F1 mice fed dehydroepiandrosterone. *J Clin Invest* 1985; 75:2091.

McCormick DL, Rao KV, Johnson WD, Bowman-Gram TA, Steele VE, Lubet RA, Kellof GJ. Exceptional chemopreventive activity of low-dose dehydroepiandrosterone in the rat mammary gland. *Cancer Res* 1996; 56(8):1724–6.

McLachlan JA, Serkin CD, Bakouche O. Dehydroepiandrosterone modulation of lipopolysaccharide-stimulated monocyte cytotoxicity. *J Immunol* 1996; 156(1):328–35.

McMichael AJ. Serum cholesterol and human cancer. *Hum Nutr* 1991; 7:141–58.

Mitchell LE, Sprecher DL, Borecki IB, Tice T, Laskarzewski P, Rao DC. Evidence of an association between DHEAS and nonfatal, premature myocardial infarction in males. *Circulation* 1994; 89:91–3.

Mulder JW, Frissen PH, Kirjnen P, et al. Dehydroepiandrosterone as predictor for progression to AIDS in asymptomatic HIV-infected men. *J Infect Dis* 1992; 165(3):413–8.

Nafziger AN, Herrington DM, Bush TL. Dehydroepiandrosterone and dehydroepiandrosterone sulfate: Their relation to cardiovascular disease. *Epidemiol Rev* 1991; 13:267–93.

Nestler JE, Clore JN, Blackard WG. Dehydroepiandrosterone: The "missing link" between hyperinsulinemia and atherosclerosis? *Faseb J* 1992; 6(12):3073–5.

Nestler JE, Barlascini CO, Clore JN, Blackard WG. Dehydroepiandrosterone reduces serum low-density lipoprotein levels and body fat but does not alter insulin sensitivity in normal men. *J Clin Endocrinol Metab* 1988; 66(1):57–61.

Okabe T, Haji M, Takayanagi R, Adachi M, Imasaki K, Kurimoto F, Watanabe T, Nawata H. Up-regulation of high-affinity dehydroepiandrosterone binding activity by dehydroepiandrosterone in activated human T lymphocytes. *J Clin Endocrinol Metabol* 1995; 80(10):2993–6.

Rana A, Habib FK, Halliday P, Ross M, Wild R, Elton RA, Chisholm GD. A case for synchronous reduction of testicular androgen, adrenal androgen and prolactin for the treatment of advanced carcinoma of the prostate. *Eur J Cancer* 1995; 31A(6):871–5.

Rasmusson KR, Arrowood MJ, Healey MC. Effectiveness of dehydroepiandrosterone in reduction of cryptosporidial activity in immunosuppressed rats. *Antimicrob Agents Chemother* 1992; 36:220–2.

Rasmussen KR, Healey MC, Cheng L, Yang S. Effects of dehydroepiandrosterone in immunosuppressed adult mice infected with Cryptosporidium parvum. *J Parasitol* 1995; 81(3):429–33.

Regelson W, Loria R, Kalimi M. DHEA—the "Mother Steroid." *Ann NY Acad Sci* 1994; 719:553–63.

Rimm EB, et al. Vitamin E consumption and the risk of coronary heart disease in men. *N Engl J Med* 1993; 328:1450.

Schwab R, Waiters CA, Weksler ME. Host defense mechanisms and aging. *Semin Oncol* 1989; 16:20–7.

Schwartz AG. Inhibition of spontaneous breast cancer formation in female C3H

(Avy/a) mice by long term treatment with dehydroepiandrosterone. *Cancer Res* 1979; 39:1129–32.

Schwartz AG, Hard GC, Pashko LL, Abou-Gharbia M, Swern D. Dehydroepiandrosterone: An antiobesity and anti-carcinogenic agent. *Nutri Cancer* 1981; 3:46–53.

Schwartz AG, Pasko L, Whitcomb JM. Inhibition of tumor development by dehydroepiandrosterone and other related steroids. *Toxicol Pathol* 1986; 14:357–62.

Spencer NFL, Poynter ME, Hennebold JD, Mu HH, Daynes RA. Does DHEAS restore immune competence in aged animals through its capacity to function as a natural modulator of peroxisome activities? *Ann NY Acad Sci* 1995; 774:200–15.

Stahl F, Schnorr D, Pilz C, Dorner G. Dehydroepiandrosterone (DHEA) levels in patients with prostatic cancer, heart disease, and under surgery stress. *Exp Clin Endocrinol* 1992; 99:68–70.

Stampfer MJ, et al. Vitamin E consumption and the risk of coronary disease in women. *N Engl J Med* 1993; 328:1444.

Stephens NG, Parsons A, Schofield P, Kelly F, Cheeseman K. Randomized controlled trial of vitamin E in patients with coronary disease: Cambridge Heart Antioxidant Study (CHAOS). *Lancet* 1996; 347:781–6.

Suzuki T, Suzuki N, Daynes RA, Engleman EG. Dehydroepiandrosterone enhances IL2 production and cytotoxic effector function of human T cells. *Clin Immunol Immunopathol* 1991; 202–11.

Suzuki T, Suzuki N, Engelman EG, Mizushima Y, Sakane T. Low serum levels of dehydroepiandrosterone may cause deficient IL-2 production of lymphocytes in patients with systemic lupus erythematosus (SLE). *Clin Exp Immunol* 1995; 99(2):251–5.

Teller MN, in *Tolerance, Autoimmunity and Aging.* MM Sigel and RA Good (eds.). Charles C Thomas, Springfield, IL, 1972, 39–52.

Van Vollenhoven RF, Engleman EG, McGuire JL. An open study of DHEA in systemic lupus erythematosus. *Arthritis Rheum* 1994; 37(9):1305–10.

Weinstein RE, Lobocki CA, Gravett S, Hum H, Negrich R, Herbst J, Greenberg D, Pieper DR. Decreased adrenal sex steroid levels in the absence of glucocorticoid suppression in postmenopausal asthmatic women. *J Allergy Clin Immunol* 1996; 97(1 Pt 1):1–8.

Wisniewski TL, Hilton CW, Morse EV, Svec F. The relationship of serum DHEAS and cortisol levels to measures of immune function in human immunodeficiency virus-related illness. *Am J Med Sci* 1993; 305(2):79–83.

Yen SS, Morales AJ, Khorram O. Replacement of DHEA in aging men and women. *Ann NY Acad Sci* 1995; 774:128–42.

Zumhoff B, Levin J, Rosenfeld RS, et al. Abnormal 24 hour mean plasma concentrations of dehydroepiandrosterone and dehydroepiandrosterone sulfate in women with primary operable breast cancer. *Cancer Res* 1981; 41:3360–3.

CHAPTER 4

DHEA, Stress, and Your Life

Not long ago researchers gave a group of graduate students a questionnaire to determine how they were handling stress. The questionnaire was designed to separate the students into two groups: those who saw college as an enjoyable challenge and those who were feeling overwhelmed.

Both groups were experiencing the same academic demands. Both had to figure out how they would pay for the next semester, who they would date, and where they would live. It's just that one group was stimulated by those challenges, while the other group was striving to cope. Sounds like life, doesn't it?

Blood tests revealed that the students who were feeling overwhelmed had *one-third* the NK cell activity of those who were enjoying the experience. Remember that NK cells are the body's primary anticancer and antiviral defense.

When I first read the study, I had the same response you probably just did. I said to myself, "*That's not fair.* Those kids need more immune strength, not less." Then I remembered that nature doesn't care a whit about you or me. Nature cares about the survival of the human race, and lowering those kids' NK cells was just its way of weeding out the folks who can't cut it. It's survival of the fittest, and that goes for emotional strength as much as for physical ability.

HOLMES AND RAHE'S
SOCIAL READJUSTMENT RATING SCALE
(A Predictor of Stress-Related Disease or Disability)

Pencil in the value of items that apply to you during the past year. Add your score and compare it with the range of scores given below the test.

EVENT	VALUE	YOUR SCORE
Death of spouse	100	____
Divorce	73	____
Marital separation	65	____
Jail term	63	____
Death of close family member	63	____
Personal injury or illness	53	____
Marriage	50	____
Fired from work	47	____
Marital reconciliation	45	____
Retirement	45	____
Change in family member's health	44	____
Pregnancy	40	____
Sex difficulties	39	____
Addition to family	39	____
Business adjustment	39	____
Death of close friend	37	____
Change to different line of work	36	____
Change in number of marital arguments	35	____
Loan over $10,000	35	____
Foreclosure of mortgage or loan	31	____
Change in work responsibilities	30	____
Son or daughter leaving home	29	____
Trouble with in-laws	29	____
Outstanding personal achievement	29	____
Spouse begins or stops work	28	____
Starting or finishing school	26	____
Change in living conditions	26	____
Revision of personal habits	25	____
Trouble with boss	24	____
Change in work hours, conditions	23	____
Change in residence	20	____
Change in schools	20	____
Change in recreational habits	20	____
Change in religious activities	19	____

EVENT	VALUE	YOUR SCORE
Change in social activities	19	___
Loan under $10,000	18	___
Change in sleeping habits	17	___
Change in number of family gatherings	16	___
Change in eating habits	15	___
Vacation	13	___
Christmas/holiday season	12	___
Minor violation of law	10	___
Your Score		___

Less than 150—37% chance of experiencing stress-related illness
150–300—51% chance of stress-related illness
More than 300—80% chance of stress-related illness

Reprinted by permission of the publisher from "The Social Readjustment Rating Scale" by TH Holmes and RH Rahe, Journal of Psychosomatic Research, Vol. II, p. 213. Copyright © 1968 by Elsevier Science Inc.

THE POWER OF STRESS MANAGEMENT

Here's the good news. When the burned-out students were given stress management training, their NK cell levels rose to normal in the course of *one semester*. This is a tremendously important lesson. It explains why researchers today can use a one-page questionnaire that measures life change and predict with uncanny accuracy whether an individual will develop a significant illness in the next year. The questionnaire, known as the Holmes and Rahe Social Readjustment Rating Scale, asks you to circle the life changes you have experienced in the last twelve months.

When Holmes and Rahe developed this test forty years ago, they didn't know about NK cells. They just knew that human beings usually have difficulty coping with change. Many changes mean more stress, and more stress means a greater likelihood of illness.

Some events from the questionnaire, such as the death of a spouse, are obviously traumatic and are weighted heavily. But note that even "good" events are listed, such as marriage, retirement, holidays, and vacations. Any activity or event that causes a readjustment of time or attention is perceived by the body as stress.

That means you and I are in deep trouble, because the amount of change we are exposed to today is astounding. As I discussed in Chapter 1, for 1.6 million years little changed but the seasons. Even in our lifetime it is easy to see how change has accelerated. My grandfather held the same job for fifty years; my father, for forty. Today the average American changes jobs every three years. You can spend years preparing for a job that becomes obsolete the day you graduate. If you look at the countless changes brought about by technology and communications, it's a wonder anyone remains healthy. But some do, and that's what we have to explore.

CHANGE WITHOUT STRESS

To say that the human mind is amazing is a profound understatement. One of the most remarkable facets of the brain is how it processes information. All day information pours into the brain from every sensory organ and is instantly compared to other information stored in more than 100 billion neurons. The part of the brain known as the hypothalamus then determines the appropriate response: "That's okay," "That needs immediate attention," or *"Panic!"*

But remember the example of the college students. The same event can be interpreted by different people in completely different ways. Did every stressed-out student have a malfunctioning hypothalamus? No. Their brains just interpreted events differently on the basis of previous information and training.

The most important factor appears to be control. When people feel they have control over a situation, they can overcome obstacles and endure stress. It's the feeling of powerlessness or the belief that the situation will never end that appears to move stress to the point of distress. This applies to everything from little annoyances to life-threatening catastrophes. Studies show, for example, that the greatest stress associated with a medical test is not the test itself or even the reporting of bad news: It's the time between the test and the availability of results. Human beings want to have a clear sense of what to do. If we lack that information or believe that no action is possible, stress becomes something else—agony, sorrow, panic, disaster.

The important point here is that *you can change the information base and responses of your brain.* They are not carved in stone. They are not genetic. They are the sum total of what you have experienced before, and you can change them through awareness and motivation.

THE ANATOMY OF STRESS

Let me raise your motivation a bit. You know that stress causes a decrease in NK cell activity. That's bad because you need those cells to survive. But that's only the tip of a truly dangerous iceberg. Here's the whole story.

When the hypothalamus presses the panic button, it stimulates the release of adrenocorticotropic hormone (ACTH) from the pituitary, which acts on the adrenals to produce stress hormones, primarily epinephrine (adrenaline) and cortisol. These hormones flood the body, enabling us to respond to the danger at hand—the well-known fight-or-flight response. The effects are listed below.

MAJOR EFFECTS OF STRESS HORMONES: THE FIGHT-OR-FLIGHT RESPONSE

1. Pupils dilate to sharpen vision.

2. Heart rate and blood pressure increase to accelerate the delivery of oxygen and fuel to the muscles and critical organs.

3. Blood flow is diverted from noncritical areas such as the gastrointestinal tract to critical areas such as the heart, skeletal muscles, and liver.

4. Liver releases glucose and fatty acids into the bloodstream. Glucose is for immediate energy; fat is needed when the fight-or-flight response lasts longer than expected.

5. Bronchial tubes dilate to maximize the exchange of oxygen and carbon dioxide.

EPISODIC VERSUS CHRONIC STRESS

The nature of stress has changed a great deal since the fight-or-flight response was developed approximately 3 million years ago. You see, stress used to be *episodic*. Everything was peachy, and then all of a sudden there was a saber-toothed tiger to deal with. The stress response was perfect for that kind of challenge because ancient men and women needed that heart-pumping adrenaline rush. Whether they fought or fled, they used up every gram of glucose and fat poured into their bloodstream by the liver. When the stress was over, it was over. But today, for the most part, stress is chronic (long-lasting), and this adrenal response is killing us.

You work hard on a project that is unfairly criticized by your boss. Suddenly your face flushes, your heart pounds, and you want to scream. But screaming is frowned upon in most offices, so you stuff the feelings of anger and frustration. In fact, sitting there at your desk, your body is going through the exact same response your ancestors experienced when faced with the tiger. Only you have nowhere to run and nothing to fight. Later that day you find yourself stuck in rush-hour traffic. Under normal circumstances you'd turn on the radio and cope, but you find yourself on edge. Pretty soon you're cursing at other drivers and triggering another fight-or-flight episode.

Most people today have lives punctuated by similar experiences. In each case, whether it's traffic, a pink slip, an abusive spouse, a missed flight, or a jam-packed schedule, the one common denominator is that no immediate action is available to relieve the stress. Over time, here's what happens.

EFFECTS OF CHRONIC STRESS

1. Your blood pressure rises. Depending on how many similar situations you have to endure, it may stay elevated, damaging the sensitive tubules of your kidneys. Ultimately, kidney function is compromised, which raises blood pressure even more, which contributes to further kidney damage, which raises blood pressure . . .

2. Since the stress response pretty much shuts down the gastrointestinal tract, your lunch turns into a toxic mass of fermenting and putrefying food. Over a period of time this distress contributes significantly to disorders such as ulcers, irritable bowel syndrome, colitis, constipation, diverticulosis, food allergy, yeast overgrowth, malnutrition, and colon cancer.

3. The glucose that is dumped into your blood goes unused, so the

body has to produce an enormous amount of insulin to handle it. In time this produces wild fluctuations in blood sugar, elevated insulin and insulin resistance, and ultimately hypoglycemia and/or diabetes. Since no muscular work is performed (and there is no metabolic need for energy), this glucose is converted to fat.

4. The fat that is dumped into your blood also goes unused, so it starts to clog your arteries.

5. Your adrenals become weakened and then exhausted. Since the adrenals contribute to the production of some 150 hormones, you can imagine the downward spiral. Your blood pressure, brain and nervous system, energy metabolism, stress management, and immunity all suffer. There is not a cell in your body that is not affected.

AND NOW THE BAD NEWS . . .

The stress response causes the adrenals to decrease the production of DHEA in favor of cortisol. We now know that the decreased NK cell activity experienced by the college students is a result of lowered DHEA.

The bad news is that you can't continue to live a stress-filled life and simply compensate with a DHEA pill. The DHEA may boost your immunity, but it will do nothing to prevent the dangerous and life-shortening scenario outlined above. The solution is to alter or revise your brain's response to stress. When that is done, you eliminate the entire cascade of adrenal-related devastation. What you need is not a pill but a comprehensive approach to stress management.

Now that the bad news is over with, let's get back to seeing how DHEA can make a positive contribution to any stress management program.

HOW DHEA HELPS LIGHTEN YOUR LOAD

DHEA and stress reduction work hand in hand, and it's not just a matter of increasing NK cell activity. DHEA, you will remember, is utilized by every tissue in the body. It even plays an important role in mind, memory, and behavior.

Today DHEA is a very hot topic among neurobiochemists. A recent study reported that the age-related decline in DHEA is a causative factor in depression among the elderly. It is likely that DHEA is also the link between stress and depression. C. Norman Shealy, M.D., Ph.D., states, "We have never seen a depressed patient with optimal levels of DHEA. And no one we've seen with optimal levels of DHEA is depressed."

Other studies have found that DHEA levels correlate directly with performance in intelligence tests that require global memory skills (utilizing memories of other times and places) rather than simple memorization by rote. Research shows that DHEA given to medical and psychiatric patients can produce significant improvements in mood, energy, libido, and memory.

A landmark study has taken this research to a new level. It's one thing to observe that people with depression have low levels of DHEA, but this group of investigators took depressed patients (male and female) and gave them enough DHEA to bring blood levels to the midnormal range of a young healthy individual. That turned out to be 30 to 90 mg per day. The result? Significant improvement in subjective and objective ratings of depression, significant improvement in verbal memory skills, and no adverse side effects. What's more, these improvements were directly proportional to the increase in DHEA levels; that is, the people who experienced the greatest increase in DHEA were the ones who improved the most.

DHEA AND SEROTONIN

DHEA has been categorized as a neurosteroid because it is metabolized directly by the brain and has a wide range of effects on brain chemistry, memory, mood, and behavior. It appears to increase serotonin levels naturally, which is something millions of Americans are currently doing artificially with drugs such as Prozac®. Preliminary evidence shows that DHEA may even help protect the brain against age-related disorders such as Alzheimer's disease.

We should be doing everything we can to maximize the production of DHEA throughout life, but most people unknowingly do the opposite. They are caught in a downward spiral of stress and decreasing DHEA that gets worse as they grow older. Have you ever noticed, perhaps when your elderly parents or grandparents were visiting, that everything is a big deal to them? What to a younger person might be an inconvenience or a minor hassle is for them an insurmountable problem. This is a well-understood degeneration of the brain that appears to be directly related to DHEA levels.

HOW TO DOUBLE YOUR DHEA, DECREASE STRESS, AND ENJOY LIFE

Sorry if this chapter has been a bit stressful so far. I'm just getting to the really good news—and it's extraordinarily good news, too. It confirms what researchers have suspected, which is that stress revision confers direct, powerful, and measurable benefits in a fairly short period. Moreover, these benefits are cumulative, contributing to an upward spiral that can enrich your life in countless ways.

No, you don't have to sit in a cave and meditate (unless you want to). Research has identified a wide range of effective techniques for any personality or lifestyle. The goal of stress revision is not to eliminate stress but to transform it.

I try not to use the phrase *stress management*. First, it creates an image of intractable pressure that is so formidable, all you can do is try somehow to *manage* it. Second, stress is not a bad thing when it leads to greater enjoyment of life or a more intense relationship with life. I know people who manage stress quite well, but I wouldn't want to spend much time with them. The people I'm attracted to incorporate a tremendous amount of stress in their lives and use it to heighten their experience and expression of passion and vitality.

I like to think in terms of transforming stress into something positive: maximizing creativity, love, and joy. If you had a script and hated the ending, you'd revise it. If you're not enjoying the script of your life, you have to understand that it can be revised, too.

Please don't think I am trivializing the pressures and tragedies life throws at us. I'm not saying that it's easy or simple to change your life. Sometimes it's incredibly difficult, but it can be done. You just need the tools.

YOGA AND MEDITATION

Research has shown that yoga and meditation can lower blood pressure, relieve anxiety, enhance overall health, accelerate weight loss, improve sleep, and increase blood levels of DHEA. There's no better place to start your stress revision program.

One of the most positive things I have done in my life is to study yoga. I have gained insight, greater health, and a significant degree of equanimity from the physical practice and meditation. The movements of yoga, like tai chi, are centering, relaxing, strengthening, and stimulating—all at the same time. With the right teacher you will experience a sense of clear awareness and peace starting with the very first class, and it gets better with practice.

Meditation is also extremely valuable. People have the idea that it's an escape from worldly cares and concerns, a kind of cosmic cocoon, but that's the Hollywood stereotype. Meditation is a very proactive practice. It will not bury or hide anything. On the contrary, it brings everything up for review. This review, however, is entirely different from your normal obsessions and fears. It is objective and calm, and there is a piercing clarity to the process that quickly brings priorities into focus.

And isn't that what we all want? We want to know what is *really* important, because life is short and we don't want to waste a single moment obsessing about stuff that is meaningless in the long run.

The most important thing for your mind is to have clear instructions, an action plan. That's the difference between coping and cracking. But that plan is sometimes impossible to see, and that's not your fault. The fact is that life today creates an information overload in our brains. Meditation can help you deal with the overload and restore your sense of clarity and purpose.

Meditation, of course, does more than help you sort things out. One of the most encouraging things I ever heard was the concept that the mind, more than anything else, desires peace. Meditation is the path to that fulfillment in that it synchronizes your actions with your core desires. The mind responds by creating the insights and awareness you need.

There are many styles and techniques of meditation. Chances are that one will be right for you, and I encourage you to "shop around." The most well-known system is transcendental meditation (TM®), and you are likely to find a number of other practices taught in your community.

MORE TOOLS FOR HEALING

Are you more likely to enjoy listening to soothing music or deep relaxation tapes? These tapes are available from a number of the sources listed in Appendix A. Special neuroacoustic tapes are also available that use specific auditory cues to bring the mind into the alpha, or relaxed, awareness state.

Interestingly, many of these tapes use primordial sounds such as ocean waves, a running stream, crickets, or wind to soothe and relax a frenzied mind. I do a great deal of traveling and always pack a portable cassette player and a few neuroacoustic tapes.

In addition, a newly discovered group of natural substances appear to "buffer" the stress response, giving people a better handle on tension, anxiety, and even physical strain. Known as *adaptogens*, they include principally ingredients found in *Eleutherococcus* (Siberan ginseng) and the herb *Schizandra*.

STRESS REVISION TRAINING

There are hundreds of organizations today that teach relaxation techniques, including biofeedback, self-hypnosis, creative visualization, and breathing exercises. One that stands out is the Institute of HeartMath (IHM) in Boulder Creek, California. This nonprofit organization conducts a considerable amount of research, much of which has been published in national and international medical journals. IHM offers an array of books and tapes and also conducts resident programs in stress revision. Just-completed breakthrough research shows that this technique (called Cut-Thru®), practiced for only one month, can result in an average 100 percent increase in DHEA and a 23 percent decrease in cortisol.

This is monumental. IHM was not the first to document improvements in the DHEA:cortisol ratio after stress management, but these are certainly the best results obtained so far. Just think: By reducing the number of stress hormones coursing through the body, a person naturally starts producing more DHEA. More DHEA means greater energy, enhanced mental and emotional health, and a whole cascade of positive effects throughout the body. This is the solution to the twentieth-century blues, a way to get back in sync with our genes and reestablish a sense of harmony and peace in our lives.

Life in the twentieth century is just too chaotic, fast-paced, and stressful. We all need proactive tools to manage change. We all need support from friends, family, and community. It has been shown that behavioral therapy to reduce feelings of isolation in the elderly can result in significant increases in DHEA. Individuals who enjoy a deep sense of community—religious, ethnic, or merely geographic— have decreased risk for heart disease and cancer. Community builds immunity.

But even if you practice stress revision techniques—even if you meditate, go for walks, listen to tapes, and stand on your head—there is still a widespread practice that is working against you and will sabotage your best efforts. It's everywhere, in your home, office, and school. It's the crutch you don't think you could live without. Can we talk?

PICK YOUR POISON

Coffee, tea, cola, chocolate—which one gets you through the day? Sometimes it seems that our entire society revolves around the consumption of these substances, and that's not a good thing. What they all have in common is the ultimate addictive ingredient—caffeine.

Look at it this way. If your doctor gave you a drug that increased your heart rate, disrupted your normal heart rhythm, made you feel hyper, increased your cortisol levels, and gave you insomnia and headaches, wouldn't you run back to that physician with your concerns? Well, caffeine does all that and more to the majority of its users.

If caffeine were up for approval by the FDA today, it would be classified as a prescription drug. The only reason it's available at the grocery store is that it's been used for such a long time by so many people. Objectivity concerning caffeine is just about impossible because 80 percent of the adult population uses it.

Reporters and editors who depend on coffee to get through the day hesitate to print research condemning caffeine, and the international coffee organizations and cola beverage companies are extremely powerful. Institutes set up to comply with FDA inquiries are controlled by the caffeine industry. Scientists who come up with damning evidence against caffeine are threatened and ostracized.

It's pure spy novel deceit, and it's all part of how you are manipulated to consume caffeine from cradle to grave. You owe it to yourself to look carefully and honestly at America's number-one drug addiction.

The Addiction of a Lifetime

In America caffeine addiction takes hold early in life. Children start out on hot chocolate, candy bars, and soft drinks. Later we graduate to coffee and spend the remainder of our lives consuming huge quantities of coffee, tea, cola beverages, diet pills, and caffeine-laced medications.

We are experiencing an incredible boom in the coffee market. Coffee shops are opening in record numbers, appearing in bookstores, hotels, laundromats, and even health food stores. Coffee is being sold from kiosks and carts, in cups, cans, and bottles. Industry forecasts predict that Americans will import more than 2.5 *billion* pounds of coffee beans in 1999.

This could have been predicted, and not only because baby boomers are running out of steam. A significant number of café customers are in their teens and twenties. What we are witnessing is a sedentary and malnourished society unable to generate the energy needed to get through the day and duped into thinking that vitality can be found in a coffee cup. But caffeine does not give you energy; *it gives you stress.*

Caffeine raises cortisol, the body's primary stress hormone, and lowers DHEA. It also decreases the panic threshold in the brain. An event or situation that could have been handled easily trips the alarm and sends us into the fight-or-flight response. Tension builds, blood pressure rises, and blood levels of glucose and fat increase. Our adrenals are so busy pumping stress hormones in response to caffeine that they aren't available to deal with other important health issues. Allergy, chronic fatigue, and autoimmune disorders all tend to be more prevalent and serious in people who consume large amounts of caffeine.

Caffeine-related side effects usually show up in the fourth and fifth decades of life. Many of my clients tell the same frightening tale of sitting at a desk in midafternoon. They've just hammered down the fourth cup of coffee, but they can hardly keep their eyes open. Their brain is fogged in, but the heart is pounding. In other words, they've reached the point where coffee no longer provides a lift; it merely jacks up the nervous system, making them feel fatigued and hyper at the same time.

Caffeine is a powerful drug. We know that it is not harmless; on the contrary, it contributes to a wide range of health disorders. If you are a regular caffeine user, chances are high that the drug is affecting the quality of your life. You probably depend on the stimulating "lift" to energize your body and clear your mind. You also may rely on the caffeine and related compounds found in pain and allergy medications. In fact, if you're like most Americans, you find it hard to get through the day without caffeine.

The Java Jolt

By far the most prevalent caffeine source is coffee. Coffee is addictive, and it has powerful side effects. If you try to kick the habit, there is a well-defined and extremely painful period of withdrawal. No wonder most people would rather do anything than give up coffee. What they don't realize is that they're substituting artificial energy for genuine vitality, and the difference between the two is like night and day.

When I ask patients about their reasons for drinking coffee, the most common response is "I need the energy." The irony is that *caffeine actually causes fatigue*. Depending on coffee for a quick boost will work for a while, but in the long run it will leave you with exhausted adrenals, decreased DHEA production, and problems regulating blood sugar.

On the mental level, caffeine puts us on a roller-coaster ride where periods of clarity are interspersed with confusion, depression, and mental lethargy. Mental alertness is not something that disappears in late adolescence. We throw it away by damaging our nervous and endocrine systems with caffeine.

Finally, on the emotional level, we need to have a sense of peace in our lives. Relationships with friends, partners, and coworkers all depend on harmony, which is destroyed by anxiety, irritability, and tension. Caffeine not only intensifies the stress in our lives but makes us less able to cope.

Flying Off the Handle

Studies show that the vast majority of coffee drinkers use regular coffee, not decaffeinated. For the purpose of this discussion we will define a cup of coffee as 6 ounces of regular drip coffee containing 90 mg of caffeine. Keep in mind that few of us drink coffee by the cup. Mugs, for example, hold 12 to 16 ounces and so represent about two and a half cups.

When I ask someone how much coffee she drinks and she says, "Oh, no more than three cups a day," I invariably find that it's three large mugs, or six cups of coffee. Then there are the *large* Styrofoam cups found in coffee shops and delis—16 to 20 ounces, or the equivalent of three cups of coffee. One of my clients told me that he drank only one cup of coffee a day. It turned out to be a giant 32-ounce convenience store mug with a vented cover for drinking while driving. That man consumed *453 mg* of caffeine on his way to work. No wonder there's so much conflict and tension at the office. Most employees are ready to blow a gasket by the time they walk in the door.

What's your daily caffeine intake? To find out, take a minute to complete the quiz on page 86. If caffeine's not a problem for you, great, but if it is, confronting the addiction is the only way to do something about it.

Your Caffeine Quotient

In the first column enter the number of servings, then multiply to get your total caffeine intake from each source. Figures given for beverages are based on one 6-ounce cup. Remember that most coffee mugs hold 12 to 14 ounces; a large Styrofoam cup holds 12 to 16 ounces. Amounts listed are averages.

The Price You Pay: Caffeinism

Health experts in the fields of endocrinology, neurology, and psychology are finally getting a picture of what they call *caffeinism*.

DAILY CAFFEINE INTAKE CHART

SERVINGS PER DAY	ITEM	CAFFEINE	TOTAL
Coffee____	Drip brewed	90 mg per cup	____
	Percolated	140 mg per cup	____
	Instant	112 mg per cup	____
	Brewed decaf	7 mg per cup	____
	Instant decaf	3 mg per cup	____
Tea____	Brewed	50 mg per cup	____
	Canned ice tea	30 mg/12 oz can	____
Cocoa____	Cocoa beverages	13 mg per cup	____
Soft drinks____	Coke (diet and regular)	33 mg	____
(12-ounce can)	Pepsi (diet and regular)	38 mg	____
	Tab	32 mg	____
	Dr Pepper	41 mg	____
	Mountain Dew	54 mg	____
	RC Cola	36 mg	____
Medications ____	Anacin	32 mg	____
(per tablet)	Dristan	16 mg	____
	Dexatrim	200 mg	____
	Excedrin	65 mg	____
	Midol	32 mg	____
	No Doz (regular)	100 mg	____
	Vivarin	200 mg	____
	Vanquish	33 mg	____
Chocolate ____	Milk chocolate	6 mg per ounce	____
	Baking chocolate	35 mg per ounce	____
	Average candy bar	20 mg per bar	____

TOTAL DAILY CAFFEINE INTAKE   ____

Encompassing a wide range of symptoms, caffeinism has been found to result from as little as 100 mg per day.

If your total is over 300 mg per day, you may have a mental and physical dependency. There is an almost 200 percent increase in the risk for ulcers and (for women) fibrocystic disease at that level. An intake of 600 mg or more indicates almost certain addiction. Research suggests that your risk of heart attack may be twice that of noncaffeine users.

If your intake is over 1,000 mg per day, you're hooked. You may need medical help to kick the habit.

LETTING GO OF CAFFEINE

Life after caffeine does not have to be dull, dreary, or lethargic. In fact, breakthrough research in human metabolism and brain biochemistry has made it possible for you to enjoy greater energy and alertness *without* caffeine than you ever experienced when you were "on" the drug. In Chapter 6 you will read about a newly discovered group of substances known as bioenergetic nutrients. They can vastly improve your metabolic efficiency and therefore the production of energy in every cell in your body.

Remember, caffeine only creates an artificial emergency that sends panic from your adrenals throughout your brain and body. Bioenergetics, in contrast, provide essential nutrients that your body needs to create energy—*real* energy. These nutrients are in very short supply in the American diet, and when tissue levels are restored, profound changes can be experienced in the way you look, feel, and experience life. It's important to note, however, that the results from bioenergetics depend to a great extent on your DHEA level. Thus, the perfect program for rejuvenation will include four important steps:

1. Learn how to destress your life. This alone can increase DHEA dramatically.

2. Use DHEA supplements if necessary to raise your levels to prime peak.

3. Optimize your body's production of energy with bioenergetics.

4. Use your newfound energy to exercise and improve your fitness level.

EFFECTS OF CAFFEINISM

Do you experience any of the following on a recurrent or frequent basis?

	YES	NO
1. Energy swings, periods of fatigue	__	__
2. Mood swings, periods of depression	__	__
3. Headaches	__	__
4. Gastrointestinal distress, cramping, diarrhea	__	__
5. Constipation	__	__
6. Premenstrual syndrome, menstrual irregularity	__	__
7. Painful and/or sensitive lumps in the breast	__	__
8. Insomnia	__	__
9. Clenching the jaw or grinding the teeth during sleep	__	__
10. Anxiety	__	__
11. Irritability, including inappropriate "fits" of anger	__	__
12. Involuntary movement in the leg (restless leg syndrome)	__	__
13. Irregular or rapid heart rate	__	__
14. Light-headedness	__	__
15. High blood pressure	__	__
16. Ulcers	__	__
17. Anemia	__	__
18. Shortness of breath	__	__
19. Difficulty concentrating and/or memory loss	__	__
20. Ringing in the ears	__	__
21. Coldness in the extremities, especially fingertips	__	__

Key: If you have five to six "yes" answers, caffeine is a problem for you. If you have seven to nine "yes" answers, caffeine is a major problem. If you have ten or more "yes" answers, your caffeine intake represents a serious health risk that may decrease your life expectancy.

GETTING OFF THE BEAN

If you've decided to see what life is like without the metabolic stress and damage from caffeine, I encourage you *not* to do it cold turkey. The withdrawal effects include almost paralyzing fatigue and splitting headaches. Better to wean yourself off the habit gradually. If you're an eight-cup-per-day person, reduce your intake by no more than one cup every few days. It should take you a few weeks to get down to two cups a day. And during this time it is best to start taking bioenergetic nutrients.

The two-cup level is an important threshold. From there to zero is the critical hurdle, and that should take you another two weeks, gradually reducing your intake or substituting decaffeinated coffee. Another strategy that works well is to substitute two cups of tea for the two cups of coffee. In fact, one or two cups of green or black tea a day appears to be quite harmless and may even confer some anti-cancer benefits.

A CLINICAL PERSPECTIVE

In over a decade of practice as a clinical nutritionist, I have seen thousands of people who suffered from the effects of caffeinism. In most cases their anxiety, headaches, insomnia, or premenstrual syndrome (PMS) could be alleviated simply by avoiding caffeine.

Those, however, were the lucky ones. Others were not so fortunate. There was the woman whose baby was born with birth defects because no one told her to avoid caffeine during pregnancy. There was the man who underwent three surgical operations and nearly had his stomach removed because his ulcers would not heal. No one told him to avoid caffeine. And what about the people misdiagnosed as neurotic or even psychotic, who spend years of their lives and small fortunes on psychotherapy—all because no one asked them about their caffeine intake?

It's well documented that one of caffeine's most debilitating long-term effects is malnutrition. Caffeine, along with theobromine and other substances in coffee, causes a loss of B vitamins, calcium, magnesium, and other minerals. Absorption of iron can be inhibited up to 85 percent when you have coffee with a meal. To make matters worse, coffee may be responsible for making you crave fats. It's another survival mechanism. Back in the Paleolithic days insufficient food intake would raise blood levels of cortisol, triggering a desire to eat fat. This makes sense; fat contains the most calories. Today, of course, you can elevate cortisol with a cup of coffee and get the same result, thus the common combination of coffee and a doughnut.

For anyone suffering from chronic illness, it makes sense to stay away from caffeine completely, especially if that illness causes fatigue and weakness. You may think coffee is helping you cope, but it's doing just the opposite and making your recovery even more difficult.

KICKING THE HABIT: CAROL'S STORY

Carol was a thirty-eight-year-old professional who was certain she could not succeed without coffee. When I suggested that coffee was a major factor in her monthly PMS, breast pain, and headaches, she told me she'd rather suffer than give up coffee.

In time I persuaded her to decrease her intake of coffee gradually and simultaneously start on bioenergetic nutrients (see Chapter 6). "If you feel like you're losing energy and stamina, let me know," I explained, assuring her that she could always go back to the coffee if she felt she needed it.

It took Carol over a month to eliminate coffee from her diet, but the benefits of decreased intake started almost immediately. She found that she was not as impatient when interacting with clients and coworkers. One colleague confessed that she had previously avoided Carol because of her "attitude problem."

Carol's client list grew, and she found that she was accomplishing more each day while working fewer hours. I explained that caffeine energy causes a great deal of "wheel spinning." It also tends to be fragmented, and while we think we're really doing a bang-up job, we are usually just doing a lot of banging around.

As of this writing, Carol has been caffeine-free for over a year. Her PMS, breast pain, and headaches disappeared more than six months ago and never returned. She looks back at her addiction and wonders how many executives, secretaries, administrative assistants, nurses, doctors, clerks, and computer operators are needlessly suffering from the same "female problems," *all addicted to the cause of their pain.*

CONCLUSION: BEATING THE STRESS EPIDEMIC

Can there be any doubt that stress has reached epidemic proportions in this country? Health experts tell us that roughly 80 percent of all doctor visits are for stress-related disorders. We know the effects of stress on the body, mind, and emotions, but sometimes it seems that we're caught in a treadmill like mice in a cage.

The treadmill analogy is not far off. While you're in it, there doesn't seem to be any escape from stress, and it's precisely that feeling of helplessness that creates the damage. How many times have you looked back at a stressful situation and seen with perfect clarity what would have been the ideal course of action? But while you were in the thick of it, all you could feel was intense anger or fear. It's those Paleolithic genes again. The dangers you are wired to deal with were episodes of immediate danger in which every ounce of energy and attention had to be mobilized to fight or flee. And here we are in the time-warp present, where stress is entirely different. It's a kettle of soup ready to boil over at any moment.

THE STRESS EPIDEMIC

- Disabling stress has doubled over the last six years.
- Seventy-two percent of American workers experience frequent stress-related physical or mental conditions that greatly increase health care costs.
- Forty percent of employee turnover is due to stress.
- One million employees per day are absent from work because of stress-related disorders.[1]

The solution is hidden in the paragraph above. First of all, turn down the heat under the kettle. That means eliminating as much of the "background" stress as you can. Get off caffeine. Get together with your family, friends, or church and develop better support systems. Trade baby-sitting with a neighbor. Reach out for help and help others whenever you can. We're all in this together.

Then take some of the soup out of the kettle. That means simplifying your life as much as you can. If you're working an extra job so you can afford a boat, ask yourself if the cost of your health and the time away from your family are worth it. If you're going crazy driving your kids all over town, ask yourself if they really need to be enrolled in twenty different activities every day of the week. Think about community. Remember that this arrangement of individual families isolated in little boxes is a brand-new development in the history of the human race, and so far as I can see, it's not working. For millennia we lived in tribal organizations in which all tasks were shared. Tribal societies today illustrate the tremendous advantage this provides not only in terms of responsibility but also in terms of time.

As I drive down the highway at night and look at the lights in all those houses, I can't help thinking that each family is struggling to make it. Each one has a mortgage, cars that break down, bills to pay, a roof to fix, and a lawn to mow. It's an incredibly inefficient way to live, especially when you realize that each one of those boxes contains the same equipment, paraphernalia, gadgets, electronics, and toys.

Community builds immunity, and I believe we can gain a great deal through cooperative efforts—not just logistical endeavors like car pools but meal sharing, walking "clubs," block parties, potluck dinners, and discussion and reading groups. We tend to come together when there is a disaster. How about coming together to prevent disasters?

Next, there's perspective. What if you had clear insight into a situation while the emergency or stress was happening? It would change everything, and this is a skill you can learn. It's one of the benefits of yoga, biofeedback, and just about any stress management tool you choose. It's the focus of the Cut-Thru technology taught at the IHM, and it is an integral part of life mastery.

Finally, of course, there's DHEA. The ironic thing is that people drink coffee to gain mental clarity when it does just the opposite. Studies confirm, for example, that memory skills *decrease* after the consumption of caffeine, primarily as a result of the constriction of blood vessels in the brain. And then, of course, caffeine lowers your DHEA level. That is the real killer, because DHEA may be the secret to maintaining mental sharpness throughout a 120-year life.

A growing body of scientific evidence shows that raising DHEA will definitely improve the mind. By enhancing the activity of a brain receptor known as N-methyl-D-aspartate (NMDA), DHEA can exert a powerful influence on learning and memory. Studies show, in fact, that a reduction in the number of NMDA receptors may be the cause of age-related decreases in learning ability, and scientists are eager to see what maintaining prime peak levels of DHEA can accomplish.

The connection between stress, health, and this incredible hormone is undeniable. As you learn to transform stress into just another experience, cortisol levels decrease and your body naturally starts producing more DHEA. The message going from your ancient DNA to your brain is this: "This organism is coping well. This is a successful experiment. Keep it going. Who knows what contribution this organism can make to the species?" Indeed, who knows?

BIBLIOGRAPHY

Arbeit ML, Nicklas TA, Frank GC, Webber LS, Miner MH, Berenson GS. Caffeine intakes of children from a biracial population: The Bogalusa Heart Study. *J Am Diet Assoc* 1988; 88(4):466–71.

Arnetz BB, Theorell T, Levi L, Kallner A, Eneroth P. An experimental study of social isolation of elderly people: Psychoendocrine and metabolic effects. *Psychosom Med* 1983; 45:395–406.

Bergeron R, de Montigny C, Debonnel G. Potentiation of neuronal NMDA response induced by dehydroepiandrosterone and its suppression by progesterone: Effects mediated via sigma receptors. *J Neurosci* 1996; 16(3): 1193–202.

Cameron OG, Nesse RM. Systemic hormonal and physiological abnormalities in anxiety disorders. *Psychoneuroendocrinology* 1988; 13(4):287–307.

Castonguay TW. Glucocorticoids as modulators in the control of feeding. *Brain Res Bull* 1991; 27(3–4):423–8.

Clementz GL, Dailey JW. Psychotropic effects of caffeine. *Am Fam Physician* 1988; 37(5):167–72.

Fava M, Littman A, Halperin P. Neuroendocrine correlates of the Type A behavior pattern: A review and new hypothesis. *Int J Psychiatry Med* 1987; 17:289–307.

Galard R, Gallart JM, Catalan R, Schwartz S, Arguello JM, Castellanos JM. Salivary cortisol levels and their correlation with plasma ACTH levels in depressed patients before and after the DST. *Am J Psychiatry* 1991; 148(4):505–8.

Gilbert SG, Rice DC, Reuhl KR, Stavric B. Adverse pregnancy outcome in the monkey (Macaca fascicularis) after chronic caffeine exposure. *J Pharmacol Exp Ther* 1988; 245(3):1048–53.

Glaser JL, Brind JL, Vogelman JH, Eisner MJ, Dillbeck MC, Willace RK, Chopra D, Orentreich N. Elevated serum dehydroepiandrosterone sulfate levels in practitioners of Transcendental Meditation (TM). *J Behav Med* 1992; 15(4):327–41.

Gustafsson O, Theorell T, Norming U, Perski A, Ohstrom M, Nyman CR. Psychological reactions in men screened for prostate cancer. *Br J Urol* 1995; 75(5):631–6.

Hermida RC, Halberg F, del Pozo F. Chronobiologic pattern discrimination of plasma hormones, notably DHEAS and TSH classifies an expansive personality. *Chronobiologia* 1985; 12:105–36.

Holmes TH, Rahe RH. The Social Readjustment Rating Scale. *J Psychosom Res* 1968; 11:213.

Hornsby P. Biosynthesis of DHEA by the human adrenal cortex and its age-related decline. *Ann NY Acad Sci* 1995; 774:29–46.

Kalimi M, Regelson W (eds.). *The Biological Role of Dehydroepiandrosterone.* Walter de Gruyter, Berlin, 1990.

Labbate LA, Fava M, Oleshansky M, Zoltec J, Littman A, Harig P. Physical fitness and perceived stress: Relationships with coronary artery disease risk factors. *Psychosomatics* 1995; 36(6):555–60.

Lee MA, Flegel P, Greden JF, Cameron OG. Anxiogenic effects of caffeine on panic and depressed patients. *Am J Psychiatry* 1988; 145(5):632–5.

Littman A, Fava M, Halperin P, Lamon-Fava S, MacLaughlin S, Pratt E, et al. Physiologic benefits of a stress: Type A behavior program for healthy middle-aged Army officers. *J Psychosom Res* 1993; 37:345–54.

Majewska MD. Actions of steroids on neuron: Role in personality, mood, stress, and disease. *Integr Psychiatry* 1987; 5:258–73.

Majewska MD. Neuronal actions of dehydroepiandrosterone: Possible roles in brain development, aging, memory and affect. *Ann NY Acad Sci* 1995; 774:111–9.

Morck TA, et al. Inhibition of food iron absorption by coffee. *Am J Clin Nutr* 1983; 37:416–20.

Mortola JF, Liu JH, Gillin JC, Rasmussen DD, Yen SS. Pulsatile rhythms of adrenocorticotropin (ACTH) and cortisol in women with endogenous depression: Evidence for increased ACTH pulse frequency. *J Clin Endocrinol Metab* 1987; 65(5):962–8.

Murray JB. Psychophysiological aspects of caffeine consumption. *Psychol Rep* 1988; 62(2):575–87.

Nottlemann ED, Susman EJ, Inoff-Germain G, Cutler GB, Loriaux DL, Chrousos GP. Developmental processes in early adolescence: Relationships between adolescent adjustment problems and chronologic age, pubertal stage, and puberty-related serum hormone levels. *J Pediatr* 1987; 110:473–80.

Rabin DS, Schmidt PJ, Campbell G, Gold PW, Jensvold M, Rubinow DR, Chrousos GP. Hypothalamic-pituitary-adrenal function in patients with premenstrual syndrome. *J Clin Endocrinol Metab* 1990; 71(5):1158–62.

Reus VI, Wolkowitz OW, Roberts E, Chan T, Turetsky N, Manfredi F, Weingartner H. Dehydroepiandrosterone (DHEA) and memory in depressed patients. *Neuropsychopharmacology* 1993; 9:66s.

Robel P, Baulieu EE. Dehydroepiandrosterone (DHEA) is a neuroactive neurosteroid. *Ann NY Acad Sci* 1995; 774:82–110.

Rosenberg L, Palmer JR, Kelly JP, Kaufman DW, Shapiro S. Coffee drinking and nonfatal myocardial infarction in men under 55 years of age. *Am J Epidemiol* 1988; 128(3):570–8.

Shealy CN. *DHEA: The Youth and Health Hormone.* Keats, New Canaan, CT, 1996, 43.

Smith GA. Caffeine reduction as an adjunct to anxiety management. *Bri J Clin Psychol* 1988; 27(3):265–6.

Van de Kar LD. Neuroendocrine aspects of the serotonergic hypothesis of depression. *Neurosci Biobehav Rev* 1989; 13(4):237–46.

Wolkowitz OM, Reus VI, Roberts E, et al. Antidepressant and cognition-enhancing effects of DHEA in major depression. *Ann NY Acad Sci* 1995; 774:337–9.

CHAPTER 5

DHEA and Women

The information presented in this book provides, to the best of my ability and knowledge, a balanced view concerning the sexes. I am careful to acknowledge cases where gender differences exist in research results or clinical experience. However, the fact remains that most researchers, doctors, and biochemists are men, and this has produced an unquestionably male-oriented health care system not only in America but worldwide.

The good news is that is changing. Even better news is that the change is coming not only from the increasing presence of women in these endeavors, but also, I believe, from a changing consciousness among men. You might expect this new thinking to originate from the reproductive health arena (Ob-Gyn). Over the years, however, significant contributions have also come from paleontology, anthropology, and genetics, the main focus of which has been to dispose of the male-centered view of human history.

WOMEN'S ROLE IN A COOPERATIVE SOCIETY

We are learning, for example, that from the dawn of the human race until recently women were the primary inventors. The first tools, it turns out, were not the weapons of men but the implements of women, which clothed, fed, and transported us through the ages. It turns out that the tribal organization of humankind, which spans 97 percent of our history—with women at the helm—was very cooperative and egalitarian. There was no such thing as "every man for him-self." We are learning that our contemporary view of society is con-structed from a male mind-set that is seriously flawed.

It's the cooperative part that intrigues me, because today men and women are expected to accomplish everything individually. At best, the nuclear family setup puts the burden of survival on a couple. To appreciate how unnatural this is, or at least how radically different it is from the way we were designed to live, think of present-day tribal societies in Africa and Asia. There, not only do women play a major role in *every* aspect of life, but that role, from dawn to dusk, is extra-ordinarily and entirely cooperative. Every task—from growing food to cooking, washing, making clothes, and child rearing—is undertaken with the assistance of a group.

I believe that this is very relevant to any discussion of twentieth-century health and wellness simply because women today are on their own. Our society promises a woman that she can "have it all" but for-gets to mention that she has to "do it all"—by herself. And while it may be nice in theory to run faster and jump higher, most women just want to accomplish more without feeling that any moment they're going to burn out or collapse.

Technology and "progress" aside, I believe that survival today is no different from what it has been for 1.6 million years. Only the pres-

---

FYI: BREAST CANCER STATISTICS

The one in nine figure commonly used as the incidence rate of breast cancer is not accurate. It's one in nine only if you assume that all women will live to the upper end of life expectancy, which is eighty-two years. Within that eighty-two-year span, in other words, one in nine women will get breast cancer. The actual risk for a woman is certainly signifi-cant but is much lower. I believe this widely reported figure has created unnecessary fear and anxiety, which are both risk factors for cancer.

sures have changed. In fact, as was discussed in Chapter 4, our pressures and challenges have *increased* as a result of the unbelievably fast pace of modern life. And the effect on women has been devastating.

WOMEN AT RISK

Today cardiovascular disease, breast cancer, and lung cancer are increasing causes of premature death in women. All three have significant stress, diet, and lifestyle factors. More telling is the fact that autoimmune disease is also increasing dramatically, and 70 to 90 percent of its victims are women. More than 75 percent of chronic fatigue patients are women, a figure that holds true for those diagnosed with depression and fibromyalgia.

There is no simple explanation for these alarming figures, but one thing is certain: Women today are experiencing unprecedented levels of stress and are facing that burden without the support systems that once enabled the human race to survive. Recently, scientific studies have been conducted to evaluate the effect of caregiving on a woman's health. These studies show that social interaction (tribal activity) is an extremely positive factor in helping a woman balance her caregiving role with her need for self-expression and health maintenance. Equally important is the ability to deal effectively with stress.

Never let a doctor tell you that you're *just* stressed. (You might point out that he or she is *just* completely and utterly out of touch with current medical knowledge.) Stress revision (my term for "stress management") is more than a matter of learning to relax. Chapter 4 presents a case for stress revision as the primary arm of preventive medicine. A number of critical factors contribute to the stress-induced breakdown of the human body and mind. Most relevant to this discussion are gender differences in adrenal strength and DHEA production.

THE DHEA GENDER GAP

Men produce approximately 30 percent more DHEA than women do. While a woman's ovaries contribute small amounts of DHEA (by conversion from other steroids), she must depend for the most part on adrenal production. What's more, ovarian failure at any age (from injury, disease, surgery, or menopause) will accelerate a decline in DHEA production.

Men, by contrast, produce a significant amount of DHEA in the testes. It's interesting to note that while men produce higher levels of DHEA, their age-related decline of DHEA is steeper. The net effect is that by age seventy men and women have roughly equal amounts of DHEA.

Meanwhile, because women must depend on their adrenals for DHEA production, it follows that adrenal stress will affect a woman to a much greater degree than it will a man. Adrenal stress comes from a number of places:

1. METABOLIC STRESSORS. These include fluctuations in blood sugar and insulin.

2. PAIN STRESSORS. Many women experience considerable pain on a monthly basis. Childbirth is in a class by itself.

3. DISEASE STRESSORS. Acute (short-lived) illness creates adrenal stress, and chronic (long-term) illness is worse, creating a vicious cycle in which weakened adrenals perpetuate the disease state.

4. DIETARY STRESSORS. Caffeine affects women to a greater extent than it affects men in terms of both the stimulant effects and the rebound depressant effects. Caffeine's stimulant effects appear to increase the risk for ulcers, panic attacks, muscle spasms, and high blood pressure. The rebound depressant effects may be responsible for caffeine's link to depression, constipation, allergy, and immune suppression. In addition, caffeine produces biochemical imbalances that contribute to birth defects, anemia, PMS, fibrocystic breast disease, and osteoporosis.

5. EMOTIONAL STRESSORS. Remember that the same event or situation can be interpreted differently by different people. DHEA levels appear to be a critical factor in this "crack or cope" phenomenon. The vicious cycle is incredible: Low DHEA decreases coping skills, which increases stress, which in turn stimulates cortisol, which then lowers DHEA, which decreases coping skills, which . . .

FOREWARNED IS FOREARMED

With the information below, you can prepare a survival strategy that will enable you to achieve optimum levels of health and wellness. By following these eight points, you'll do wonders to boost your body's levels of DHEA, and you'll feel and look better than you ever thought possible.

1. DON'T SMOKE. The tobacco companies' target market for the past twenty years has been women. The operative word here is *target*. Cigarettes are killing women in unprecedented numbers, and a woman who smokes ten cigarettes a day is 50 percent more likely to get lung cancer as a result compared with a man.

2. DON'T DRINK EXCESSIVELY. Alcohol damages a woman's body faster and more severely than it damages a man's body. What is moderate drinking for the man in your life may be excessive for you. Be sensitive to this difference when you share a bottle of wine at dinner. Most experts agree that one glass of wine is tolerable for a 120-pound woman. More than that will increase her risk for a number of acute and chronic disorders.

3. KEEP MOVING. Get in sync with your genes through exercise. As it turns out, physical activity is incredibly important for women. A recent twenty-year study of women age thirty-eight to sixty found that occupations including moderate activity could reduce mortality (your risk of dying) by two-thirds. Even moderate *leisure* activity reduced mortality by nearly half. Most important, this study found that women who were moderately active but then became sedentary *doubled* their mortality risk compared with women who kept moving. See Chapter 7 for valuable exercise tips.

4. EAT LIKE A CAVEWOMAN. When you review Chapter 9, you'll see what I mean by this. For most women it means eating smaller but more frequent meals and eating more fruits and vegetables. I know that time is always a big factor when it comes to meals, but salad bars can be found just about everywhere, and they offer a quick and easy way to "graze." Just be sure to avoid the prepared dishes, such as potato salad, coleslaw, and desserts.

Then there's the fiber factor to consider. Your Paleolithic ancestors consumed somewhere between 40 and 80 grams of fiber per day. Most Americans get 10 to 15 grams, and the U.S. Department of Health, the National Cancer Institute, and the American Heart Association all recommend at least 20 grams. I suggest 30 to 40 grams

---

THE FAST-FOOD TRAP[1]

You're in a rush, looking for a fast-food restaurant. You select Mexican food because you've heard that beans and rice are better than deep-fried chicken and burgers. What's more, you get a charge of self-righteous pride when you order a taco salad. (Salad, right? How bad can it be?) Well, at one national chain, it's the fattiest thing on the menu: a whopping 900 calories and 62 grams of fat!

What are the culprits? The taco shell and the dressing. If you must have the taco salad, don't eat the shell and ask for the dressing on the side.

---

because that is the level of intake most likely to reduce your risk for breast and colon cancer. You'll find some easy fiber tips in Chapter 8.

5. TAKE YOUR VITAMINS. Nutritional supplements can provide remarkable protection for women. For example, your risk of cardiovascular disease can be cut almost in half by taking 200 to 400 IU of vitamin E per day. The U.S. Department of Health is begging women of childbearing age to take a daily dose of 400 mcg of folic acid, but I would extend that advice to women of any age. After all, this level of intake not only will cut the risk of birth defects but also has been shown to have anticancer and cardiovascular benefits.

THE ROLE OF DIET IN DEGENERATIVE DISEASES

Breast cancer, prostate cancer, coronary heart disease, and colon cancer belong to the so-called Western diseases and a general opinion is that diet is a significant or even the main factor increasing incidence and mortality of these diseases in the Western world.[2]

Both vitamin E and folic acid can be obtained from a good multi-vitamin, but I would add a wide-spectrum antioxidant as well as bioenergetics and comprehensive bone, joint, and ligament support (see Chapter 9).

6. AVOID STIMULANTS. Aside from the fact that caffeine and herbal stimulants raise stress hormone levels, decrease DHEA, and damage your adrenals, there are important reasons for women to avoid the stimulant trap. Millions of women suffer from monthly or chronic pain associated with benign breast lumps. The cause of this condition, known as fibrocystic (or cystic) breast disease, has not been confirmed, but research has identified stimulants as a major contributing factor.

In 1979, Dr. John Minton of the Ohio State University College of Medicine discovered that women with this condition have abnormally high levels of a chemical messenger known as cyclic adenosine monophosphate (cAMP) in their breast tissue. Since caffeine is known to increase cAMP, Minton conducted an experiment to see whether avoidance of caffeine would help. It did. In fact, 82 percent of the women who strictly avoided caffeine experienced complete disappearance of breast lumps. In case you're wondering, cystic breast disease *does* increase the risk for breast cancer.

Encouraged by Minton's work, other researchers looked for connections between caffeine, cAMP, and PMS. Data collected from 295 college sophomores revealed a strong association between the consumption of caffeine beverages (including soft drinks) and the presence and severity of PMS. You'll find a complete discussion of the coffee quandary in Chapter 4, but let me summarize here the specific reasons for a woman to get off caffeine:

FACT: Iron deficiency, inadequate calcium intake, osteoporosis, and depression are devastating problems for women.
FACT: Caffeine dramatically reduces iron absorption.
FACT: Caffeine increases calcium loss and the risk of osteoporosis.
FACT: Caffeine produces short-term mood elevation but contributes to rebound depression.

CAFFEINE BY ANY OTHER NAME

Most people don't know that caffeine is found in plants other than the coffee bean. Tea contains caffeine (about 20 to 40 mg per cup). Guarana, a South American herb, may contain up to 10 percent pure caffeine, making it more potent than coffee. Maté, bissy nut, kola nut, cocoa, and gotu kola are all sources of caffeine. In addition, numerous herbs possess stimulant effects very similar to caffeine. Ephedra (also known as ma huang or epitonin), fo ti, and sarsaparilla are all central nervous system stimulants.

7. GET MORE SLEEP. A client of mine went backpacking for a week and came back a new woman. What do you think made the difference? She was always an avid cyclist, bicycling about 60 miles a week, so it wasn't the exercise or fresh air. It was the fact that there was no TV. When the sun went down, she went to sleep, as women have done for millions of years. No talk shows, no late-night movies. The extra sleep literally transformed her, and she vowed never again to fall into the habit of ending the day in front of the television.

Sleep is the body's rest and rejuvenation time, but so many women shortchange themselves and try to get by on five or six hours. Scientific studies show that eight or nine hours is optimal and that getting adequate sleep helps restore levels of DHEA.

Certainly children cut into sleep time, and there's no getting away from that. But if it's TV, a novel, or insomnia that's keeping you from sleeping, try these sleep aids:

- Don't use alcohol to "wind down" at the end of the day. One glass of wine with dinner should be okay, but excess alcohol alters sleep patterns. Typically, if you drink more than that, you will have no trouble getting to sleep but will tend to awaken frequently throughout the night.
- Exercise regularly throughout the day to tire your muscles but don't exercise too close to bedtime. Exercise can have an energizing effect, which is counterproductive to your body's natural process of getting ready for sleep.
- Don't smoke. (Sound familiar?) You might think that a cigarette will help you get to sleep, but smokers spend less time in both the deep restoring level of sleep and mind-restoring rapid eye movement (REM) sleep. Also, smoking in bed can be highly dangerous!
- Take a bath before bed. The water temperature should be warm

but not overly hot. Fill up the tub and add your favorite bath oil, gel, or bubbles. Give yourself a few extra minutes to soak and relax—fifteen to twenty minutes is ideal. Both your muscles and your mind will unwind with this ritual.

- Get physical. It's a myth that only men fall asleep after sex. Your body experiences a natural relaxation response after sex that leads straight to slumberland.
- Try a deep relaxation technique or audiotape. Tapes that include the sounds of nature are the most restful, as described in Chapter 4. See Appendix A for a list of sources for these tapes.
- Use a very small dose (starting at 1.5 mg) of melatonin. If melatonin proves to be of value (and it probably will), see if you get the same benefits by using it every other night.

8. OPTIMIZE YOUR DHEA PRODUCTION WITH STRESS REVISION TECHNIQUES. This is the most critical point of all. Unless you are able to alleviate stress, your body's youth-restoring DHEA will be in a constant tug-of-war with cortisol. To the degree that cortisol wins, you will age faster, look older, and suffer more serious illnesses.

After reading Chapter 4, you know that the choice is yours. It seldom *feels* that way, because so much of the time we believe that our lives are controlled by circumstances or fate. It might be wise to take a mental and emotional "inventory" and see if your mindset is one of possibility or helplessness. The Social Readjustment Scale in Chapter 4 is a good place to start. If you find that an attitude of hopelessness predominates in your life, it may be time to seek help.

I can't tell you where that help might come from, but I believe very strongly that "when the student is ready, the teacher appears." In other words, when you make a firm commitment to change, you will be guided to the appropriate avenue for help, whether it be a friend, book, church group, or therapist. The important thing is to ask.

Some women will take this inventory and conclude that they are possibility-oriented people. Being possibility-oriented does not mean that you are immune to stress, only that you are better equipped at the moment to take steps to transform stress from an enemy to a friend.

TWO EXERCISES FOR THE STRESS-DEPENDENT

Finally, there are women who believe that stress is a necessary evil. They feel that if they took steps to manage stress, they'd become less effective or less successful. To them I suggest two simple exercises.

The first can be done in less than a minute. Hold this book with one hand and clench your fist with the other hand as tightly as you can. As you read, continue to hold the fist tightly, and don't let go for about thirty seconds. When you finally release the tension in the fist, your forearm muscle will be tired and may even hurt.

That's the effect of thirty seconds of tension on one muscle. There are instruments that can measure muscle contraction, and we know that stress can produce a similar level of tension in a number of muscles, most notably the trapezius, which runs from the middle of your back, over the tops of your shoulders, and up the back of your neck. The abdominal muscles are also notable tension accumulators.

If your arm got tired holding a fist for thirty seconds, imagine how much energy you expend by holding on to stress for ten or fifteen hours a day. Stress drains your batteries. It uses up a tremendous amount of energy and accomplishes absolutely nothing. Think of what you could do with all that energy, how much more productive and successful you could be.

The second exercise takes a bit longer. Find a stress transformation technique that appeals to you: yoga, meditation, biofeedback, or any of the resources listed in Appendix A. Really apply yourself to that course or practice for thirty days and then look at your career and your relationships. See if you have become a more effective person and observe whether your feelings regarding your body and your life have changed. Ask your family members and friends if they see any change and if they like what they see. Then, if you want, you can always abandon the technique and get your stress back.

Today we tend to equate power with tension and aggression. Through stress revision you will discover that the truth is exactly the opposite. Personal power comes from vitality, from the experience of a calm, clear mind and a vibrantly healthy body. You cannot buy these qualities, but you can decide to acquire them. You can decide that you are worth the investment in time and attention, because life is short and this isn't a dress rehearsal.

WHAT ABOUT DHEA SUPPLEMENTS?

Stress revision will increase your DHEA level considerably, but if testing shows that you have not reached prime peak, you may want to take a DHEA supplement. At this point you will be faced with a mountain of conflicting information.

A common opinion is that women should not take DHEA because it will be converted to testosterone. This makes absolutely no sense. The conversion of DHEA to testosterone is natural to a woman's physiology; the levels of *both* hormones decline steeply with age. In fact, a woman of forty will have a testosterone level approximately half of what she was producing when she was twenty. That's a problem because testosterone is your power hormone. Typically, it increases feelings of competence and strength. It also increases libido—not just the desire for sex but the desire for life.

Clinical trials with women showed that testosterone increased significantly with a moderately high dose of 50 mg of DHEA per day, but the hormone was raised only to the level normally seen in a healthy young woman.

And what is the goal? Not to masculinize women but to restore DHEA and testosterone levels to the female prime peak. What are the advantages? Consider that the same 50 mg per day produced a marked increase in IGF-1, the body's repair and rebuild hormone. That may be the single most important metabolic advantage, giving a woman greater physical ability through increased muscle tone and improved protein synthesis for tissue repair. The end result of this study was a remarkable increase in perceived physical and psychological well-being among 84 percent of the women taking DHEA.

Another false alarm is that DHEA supplements will elevate estrogen levels enough to increase the risk for breast cancer, but this is unfounded. Certainly there is clinical evidence that high-dose administration may be cause for concern, but even 1,600 mg per day only doubled estrone and estradiol. A sensible approach is to start with a low dose of 10 to 25 mg of DHEA and slowly increase to a maximum of 50 mg. At that dose studies show that estrone and estradiol levels are *unchanged*.

MEDICAL BENEFITS OF DHEA

There is just not enough information to know with certainty the full range of medical benefits of DHEA. We do know that maintaining DHEA at prime peak will strengthen bones and decrease the risk for osteoporosis. Together with bioenergetics (see Chapter 6), prime peak levels of DHEA will optimize energy production, and that energy will not be limited to skeletal muscles. Energy will also go to the brain, nervous system, immune system, and adrenals. In scientific terms these functions are up-regulated to a higher level of efficiency and power. You can see the upward spiral of capability increasing action, action producing strength, strength producing confidence, confidence improving attitude, and attitude changing lives. With DHEA, it can be done.

As far as the treatment of specific diseases, you will have to work out a plan with your physician. A growing number of doctors are using DHEA with their patients, and DHEA is finally being discussed at medical conferences. The problem is that since DHEA is not being promoted by a drug company, there is no easy way for a physician to get accurate and clinically relevant information. Thus, I suggest that they use a computer-linked service specifically for doctors such as Physicians-On-Line®.

For the patient, I suggest trying to find a doctor with a track record of using DHEA with women. The best way to do this is to contact one of the laboratories listed in Appendix A. They will be happy to refer you to a physician in your area.

THE MICRONIZED VERSUS CRYSTALLINE CONTROVERSY

Today there are a number of options for the administration of DHEA. Investigators have found that a 300-mg oral dose of pure crystalline DHEA will raise testosterone above the female prime peak. This can also produce masculinizing effects such as facial hair and even voice changes.

However, micronization of that material (reducing the particle size to less than 10 μm) appears to provide the same increase in

DHEA but may have the advantage of reducing the subsequent conversion to testosterone. Finally, DHEA administered by a vaginal sup-
pository increased DHEA but *not* testosterone. This is new
information, and its clinical significance is unclear. Only a physician
can evaluate its meaning for you, taking into consideration your
medical history, present condition, and therapeutic goals. Micronization is irrelevant to the vast majority of women, who will need no
more than 20 to 50 mg of DHEA.

PHYSICIANS ON DOSAGE

In general, the clinicians I spoke with do not see a problem with supplemental DHEA in amounts from 10 to 25 mg per day. Still, Dr.
Michael Rosenbaum of Corte Madera, California, has his female
patients test their hormone levels frequently and offers the following
caveats: Start with a low dose of 5 mg and gradually increase to 25 mg
per day. Watch for any adverse effects, such as the following:

- Irritability, nervousness, or unusual feelings of anger
- Acne
- Breast swelling or tenderness
- Changes in the menstrual cycle

Jesse Hanley, M.D., the medical director of Malibu Health and
Rehabilitation in Malibu, California, has been prescribing DHEA for
five years with remarkable results. She says, "I've seen many of my
patients with CFIDS, Crohn's disease, fibromyalgia, adult onset allergies, average adult fatigue or burnout, and weak digestion—to mention a few ailments—heal deeply with DHEA administered to keep
within physiologic blood levels. I use a dose from 5 to 50 mg per day
and check blood levels every three to six months depending on the
condition and response. I also check liver functions and free testosterone levels every six to 12 months."

Dr. Hanley adds, "On numerous occasions, I have seen patients
whose natural DHEA levels started to rise after one to two years of
feeling good. These people began to require less and less DHEA supplementation. I believe this may be the result of adrenal healing."

A NEW LOOK AT "FEMALE PROBLEMS"

I am painfully aware of the tendency of males to dismiss women's problems as "hormonal," but the fact is that hormones play an important role in the way all of us experience life. We know that hormones, including DHEA, have profound neurological activity. They affect mood, memory, and behavior. Hormones exert a powerful influence on the foods we select and then determine the metabolic fate of those calories (whether they are converted to energy, muscle, or fat).

When you wake up in the morning, hormones influence your state of mind, and that sets the tone for the day, for your unfolding life. All this is undeniable. It is what we *do* with this information that makes the difference. If we make generalizations about "female problems" and respond merely by writing prescriptions, I am convinced that we as a society are doomed. That path is well marked by current suffering and frightening projections.

Imagine that you get into your car and turn the key, and all you hear is a terrible grinding noise. You have it towed to a repair shop and take a cab to work. In midmorning the mechanic calls, and the conversation goes something like this: "Ms. Jones, I have good news. We found the trouble." "Really, what is it?" "Your car won't start."

That's where we are right now in terms of women's health. Most women are aware that their present experience of wellness and fulfillment isn't working, but unless you know *why* something isn't working, you can't fix it. I believe the Paleolithic perspective opens a door of hope because it takes into account the microscopic strands of genetic material deep within your cells known as DNA. Understanding that powerful influence enables us to take steps to synchronize our genes with our behavior, and that sets in motion something I call the *alignment principle*.

THE ALIGNMENT PRINCIPLE

If you had a half dozen spools and wanted to shine a light through them from one end to the other, you would align the holes to create an unblocked path. Women have been adjusting the "spools" of their lives for decades: the physical, mental, emotional, and spiritual components that make us who we are. But there is one component that has not been recognized and therefore remains out of alignment, and that is your DNA.

You see, you are not just a physical, mental, emotional, and spiritual being that exists here in the present. You have another dimension, and that is the ancient genetic code that lies deep within your cells, responding to stress in the same way that it has for 1.6 million years. I believe that correcting the stress-induced misalignment of cortisol and DHEA will be the last critical step for women.

Using the spool analogy, you can see that until *all* the spools are aligned, it doesn't matter how many you have right. The one that is out of line will prevent the light from passing through. With stress revision and prime peak levels of DHEA, the light of vitality and well-being will finally have a chance to shine more brightly in women's lives.

BIBLIOGRAPHY

Adlercreutz H. Western diet and Western diseases: Some hormonal and biochemical mechanisms and associations. *Scand J Clin Lab Invest Suppl* 1990; 201:3–23.

Auerbach JD, Figert AE. Women's health research: Public policy and sociology. *J Health Soc Behav* 1995; Spec No:115–31.

Becker RC. Education and clinical research issues in women's health. *Cardiology* 1995; 86(4):270–1.

Bergman E, Sherrard D, Massey L. Effects of dietary caffeine intake on calcium metabolism and bone turnover in adult women. *Fed Proc* 1987; 46:632.

Cancer Facts and Figures: 1991. American Cancer Society, 1599 Clifton Road, N.E., Atlanta, GA 30329.

Casson PR, Straughn AB, Umstot ES, Abraham GE, Carson SA, Buster JE. Delivery of dehydroepiandrosterone to premenopausal women: Effects of micronization and nonoral administration. *Am J Obstet Gynecol* 1996; 174(2):649–53.

Casson PR, Faquin LC, Stentz FB, Straughn AB, Andersen RN, Abraham GE, Buster JE. Replacement of dehydroepiandrosterone enhances T-lymphocyte insulin binding in postmenopausal women. *Fertil Steril* 1995; 63(5):1027–31.

Christiansen D. Variety of fiber products protect against breast cancer. Medical Tribune News Service, July 2, 1996.

Cumming DC, Rebar RW, Hopper BR, Yen SS. Evidence for an influence of the ovary on circulating dehydroepiandrosterone sulfate levels. *J Clin Endocrinol Metab* 1982; 54:1069–71.

Ginter E. Health status in Europe and its projection up to the year 2000: II. The female population. *Cas Lek Cesk* 1996; 135(1):3–7.

Lissner L, Bengtsson C, Bjorkelund C, Wedel H. Physical activity levels and changes in relation to longevity: A prospective study of Swedish women. *Am J Epidemiol* 1996; 143(1):54–62.

Liu CH, Laughlin GA, Fischer UG, Yen SS. Market attenuation of ultradian and circadian rhythms of dehydroepiandrosterone in postmenopausal women: Evidence for a reduced 17,20 desmolase enzymatic activity. *J Clin Endocrinol Metab* 1990; 71:900–6.

London SJ, et al. A prospective study of benign breast disease and risk of breast cancer. *JAMA* 1992; 267:941–4.

Minton JP, Foecking MK, et al. Response of fibrocystic disease to caffeine withdrawal and correlation of cystic nucleotides with breast disease. *Am J Obstet Gynecol* 1979; 135:157–8.

Moen P, Robison J, Dempster-McClain D. Caregiving and women's well-being: A life course approach. *J Health Soc Behav* 1995; 36(3):259–73.

Morck TA, et al. Inhibition of food iron absorption by coffee. *Am J Clin Nutr* 1983; 37:416–20.

Slaga TJ. Critical events and determinants in multistage skin carcinogenesis, in *Carcinogenicity and Pesticides*. American Chemical Society, Washington, DC, 1989.

Tinker L. The Women's Health Initiative: Be part of the answer! (interview). *J Am Diet Assoc* 1995; 95(12): 1375.

Yen SS, Morales AJ, Khorram O. Replacement of DHEA in aging men and women: Potential remedial effects. *Ann NY Acad Sci* 1995;774:128–42.

Zumoff B, Strain GW, Miller LK, Rosner W. Twenty-four-hour mean plasma testosterone concentration declines with age in normal premenopausal women. *J Clin Endocrinol Metab* 1995; 80(4):1429–30.

CHAPTER 6

Beyond DHEA: Overcoming Fatigue, Protecting Your Joints, and Building Your Bones

By now it should be clear that aging does not proceed in a predictable, linear fashion, even though it may seem to when we look at charts depicting how our tissues and organs decline. In reality, there is always a "scatter" phenomenon, which means that plenty of people are more youthful than the norm while others age too rapidly.

The question is, What are the healthy, youthful people doing right? The answer is unequivocal: They stay active. Regular exercise of the body and mind does wonders for longevity, and this is why the DHEA Plan places so much emphasis on mental and physical "movement."

I have presented the concept of maintaining high DHEA levels to make your cells believe you are twenty-five years old again. The same can be said of maintaining appropriate levels of mental activity and exercise. While the fundamental mechanism of aging is a secret held deep within a tiny strand of DNA, we do know this much: You have a "use it or lose it" body and a "use it or lost it" mind.

In conjunction with your efforts to increase your natural levels of DHEA and supplement them when needed, you can improve your capacity for physical and mental activity even further through bioenergetics and connective tissue support. These two wonderful additions to the DHEA Plan can actually *increase* your tolerance for and enjoyment of exercise, helping you realize your full potential for optimum health and longevity.

THE BIOENERGETIC BOOST

"I just don't have the energy." How many times have you said that? We all have put off sex, exercise, playing with the kids, and a hundred other activities with the defense "I just don't have the energy."

When this statement follows a period of strenuous exercise or hard physical labor, it makes sense, but many people experience fatigue even when there is no physical reason. Doctors hear constantly from patients who arrive home at the end of the day feeling exhausted when all they did was sit at a desk. Until recently doctors would run through a battery of tests to rule out a disease-related cause and then announce, "Well, Mr./Mrs. Jones, you're just getting older."

After hearing from hundreds of these people in my clinical nutrition practice, I started searching for a better reason for unexplained fatigue. After all, there is no reasonable scientific support for the assertion that growing older causes a lack of vitality. I believe this response is common simply because doctors also feel tired. Whenever a condition is so widespread, we have a tendency to write it off as "normal."

The experience of fatigue in the absence of disease or strenuous work is not normal, and you don't have to "learn to live with it." Research has uncovered a group of natural substances that are essential for the body's production of energy. Known as *bioenergetics*, these substances have been found to be in short supply in the American diet. The result: low-efficiency metabolism, fatigue, poor exercise tolerance, and mood and energy swings. Also, bioenergetic nutrient insufficiencies make losing and maintaining weight an endless struggle.

VITAL BIOENERGETIC NUTRIENTS: THE SUPER SIX

My experience with bioenergetics began when I was invited to advise the American Olympic track and field team in 1984. At that time, the Eastern European competitors reportedly were using performance-enhancing drugs, and I was asked to find a safe and natural alternative for the U.S. athletes.

My database search covered over fifty thousand scientific and medical journals published worldwide and took me to several countries, where I spoke with nutrition and sports performance experts. Gradually, I identified six vital nutrients that are the keys to metabolic efficiency.

Each of these nutrients is required for the efficient production of energy in the body. When they are present at optimal levels, the body produces all the energy you need to work, play, and enjoy life. The six nutrients needed to fuel the energy cycle are:

• **ALPHA-KETOGLUTARIC ACID (AKG)** Although it sounds like something from a chemist's lab, AKG is an essential nutrient found in every cell of the human body. As a vital component of the energy-producing cycle, AKG levels help determine the body's metabolic efficiency. In a study with human volunteers, supplementation with AKG resulted in enhanced oxygen delivery and improved exercise tolerance. AKG is also required for the optimal metabolism of carbohydrates, fats, and proteins.

• **VITAMIN B$_6$** Vitamin B$_6$ is another key metabolic nutrient necessary for both aerobic and anaerobic energy production. Vitamin B$_6$ is also a building block for numerous biochemicals, including the enzyme needed to produce DHEA, and plays an important role in carbohydrate metabolism. This vitamin is one of the nutrients most likely to be destroyed by food processing or high-heat cooking, and insufficiency is common. The combination of vitamin B$_6$ and AKG has been shown to decrease the accumulation of lactic acid in working muscles. Since lactic acid contributes to the muscle soreness that causes many people to stop exercising, optimizing levels of these nutrients can make exercise easier and more enjoyable.

• **COENZYME Q10** This essential nutrient is needed for cellular respiration. Every cell of your body, from the top of your head to the tips of your toes, breathes—not just your lungs. Energy is produced when oxygen is combined with fuel derived from food. This biochemical "combustion" is sparked by coenzyme Q10 (CoQ10), a vitally important companion nutrient to DHEA.

CoQ10 is normally obtained from a group of nutrients known as *ubiquinones* that are often eliminated or destroyed in a highly processed diet. One group of researchers examined the level of coenzyme Q10 in obese patients and discovered a significant deficiency in over half the subjects. What's more, CoQ10 levels tend to decrease rapidly with age. A sixty-five-year-old has only 20 percent of the CoQ10 he or she had in his or her prime.

That may not be the only parallel to DHEA. Both nutrients appear to be extremely effective in reducing the risk for heart disease. In fact, CoQ10 doubles as a powerful antioxidant that works with vitamin E to prevent the oxidation of cholesterol in the blood, minimizing the damage done to arteries by the production of free radicals. What's more, the heart muscle itself is the largest user of CoQ10 of any tissue in the body, and research has demonstrated that heart CoQ10 levels correspond directly to the health of that organ.

Like DHEA, CoQ10 is essential for the proper functioning of the immune system. When explaining this to my students, I remind them that this bioenergetic nutrient can enhance energy production *throughout* the body, not just in the muscles. That means more energy for the immune system, leading researchers to classify CoQ10 as a primary immunomodulating agent.

• **CHROMIUM** Chromium's importance in bioenergetic nutrition stems primarily from the cofactor role it plays with the hormone insulin. Since insulin is required for the delivery of fuel to brain and muscles, insufficient chromium can contribute to fatigue and low metabolic efficiency. Research conducted by the U.S. Department of Agriculture found that 90 percent of the people studied were obtaining inadequate levels of chromium in the diet.

Again, there is a powerful DHEA-chromium connection. Both can help correct the metabolic defect known as *insulin resistance*, which contributes to diabetes and heart disease (see Chapter 3). Both have been shown to help lower blood cholesterol, and both can help reduce the incidence of atherosclerotic plaques.

In fact, restoring optimum levels of chromium can help increase the amount of DHEA that is available to your body. Hyperinsulinism, a condition of excessive insulin production (see Chapter 3), can be eliminated by correcting a chromium deficiency. That in turn will naturally raise DHEA levels.

Research also suggests that chromium can improve the fat-burning efficiency of weight-loss diets. Without adequate chromium, glucose tolerance (the ability to metabolize carbohydrates efficiently) is decreased. This can contribute to mood and energy swings as well as abnormal food and sugar cravings. Optimizing chromium levels is essential for maintaining a sense of control and comfort on a weight-loss program.

• **POTASSIUM AND MAGNESIUM ASPARTATE** More than thirty years of research supports the use of potassium and magnesium aspartate as antifatigue agents. Like AKG, these mineral and aspartic acid complexes appear to enhance vitality by improving the efficiency of the energy production cycle. These minerals are also essential for cardiovascular health and muscle contraction.

THE UPWARD SPIRAL

I used bioenergetics with Olympic and professional athletes to help maintain peak performance but soon realized that these nutrients could help anyone. I began to see that there was a strong similarity between a physically exhausted athlete and an inactive person with low metabolic efficiency. Both individuals are starved for oxygen and fuel: athletes because they use up energy reserves and inactive people because their bodies stop making the enzymes necessary to tap into those reserves.

Remember, your body will produce only as much energy as you require it to produce. A sedentary lifestyle lowers metabolic efficiency, leaving many people incapable of regular exercise. Bioenergetics can help change that.

The same substances I used to help athletes shave a few minutes or seconds from their performance times can give you more energy to apply to everyday life. Once you feel more energetic, you will enjoy exercise more . . . which starts a positive cycle, or upward spiral, that leads to ever-greater levels of fitness.

VITALITY SELF-EVALUATION

If you're wondering whether you need to supplement your diet with bioenergetics, the following self-evaluation can help you determine your level of energy and vitality.

Exercise frequency (weekly)	0–1	2–4	5+
Exercise intensity	easy	medium	hard

Exercise duration			
(minutes)	10–15	15–30	30+
Feelings after exercise	exhausted	tired	invigorated
Caffeine intake (weekly)			
cups of coffee/tea	4+	2–3	0–1
caffeine sodas	4+	2–3	0–1
Energy level generally	low	medium	high
Energy slumps			
(especially after lunch)	frequently	sometimes	never
Alert on awakening	never	sometimes	often
Sugar cravings	frequently	sometimes	never
Ability to cope with stress	low	medium	high
Clarity of mind	low	medium	high
Consistency of energy	erratic	medium	good

If many of your responses were in columns 1 or 2, you will probably feel a definite improvement in your energy level if you add bioenergetics to your diet.

BIOENERGETICS AND WEIGHT LOSS

In 1994 I participated in a clinical study evaluating factors that could help people achieve and maintain their ideal weight. The focus was on a permanent solution to the weight-loss struggle, and that meant we had to find a way to help people develop a higher level of fitness.

We gave a formulation of bioenergetic nutrients to the participants in this study, and the results were impressive. Subjects taking the formulation reported higher and more consistent energy, loss of food and sugar cravings, greater tolerance and enjoyment of exercise, and a feeling of "being in control." All this helped accelerate weight loss naturally and effortlessly.

For many people in the study, this was the first time they had been able to stick to a regular exercise program. For some, it was the first time they had been able to exercise and feel good afterward. People started reporting a "craving" for exercise. They said they were sleeping better and waking up more alert and optimistic.

The best news is that all these effects came from a natural approach to greater vitality. Bioenergetic nutrients help the body fulfill its inherent potential for vitality and strength. This is very different from the common approach of using caffeine and other stimulants as energy boosters. I like to think of it as the difference between beating a horse (giving it stimulants) and feeding it (providing missing nutrients).

With bioenergetics you feel natural, consistent energy instead of the frenzied or jittery feeling you get from stimulants. You may miss the instant "kick in the pants" from caffeine or other stimulants, but as your tissue levels of bioenergetics are maximized, you will experience a genuine and lasting improvement in your sense of well-being and vitality.

HOW TO ADD BIOENERGETICS TO YOUR LIFE

Because most bioenergetic nutrients are processed out of our foods, it's almost impossible to get optimal quantities even in a healthy diet. The easiest way to add bioenergetics to your life is through supplements, which you can find at health food stores. The daily doses recommended for the greatest bioenergetic benefits are as follows:

Alpha-ketoglutaric acid (AKG)	200–400 mg
Vitamin B_6	15–20 mg
Coenzyme Q10	30–40 mg
Chromium	200–300 mcg
Potassium/magnesium asparate	200–400 mg

Combining bioenergetics with a regular exercise program can dramatically improve your metabolic efficiency and make much more energy available to you. Chapter 7 will show you how to easily add regular, consistent exercise to your daily routine.

CONNECTIVE TISSUE SUPPORT: WHAT IT IS AND HOW TO GET IT

All across America, Thanksgiving is a time when grown men hurt themselves playing touch football. Either before or after the biggest dinner of the year the men of the family go out for a game while their

REPORTED BENEFITS FROM BIOENERGETIC NUTRIENTS

FOR MEN:
- No midafternoon slumps
- Increased productivity
- Greater stamina
- Improved endurance

FOR WOMEN:
- Greater and more consistent energy
- Decreased mood and energy swings
- Improved exercise tolerance
- Accelerated weight loss

wives cringe, knowing what comes next: bruises, sprains, and achy joints after falls on the hard November ground.

These episodes are common when middle-aged men act as they did in their twenties. For twenty-year-olds falling on the frozen earth is no big deal, since their high muscle mass protects their joints, but for most forty-year-olds it's a different story. Loss of muscle decreases joint protection, and extra fat increases joint stress. Moreover, tendons and ligaments become less flexible as we age, and all this increases the risk of injury.

DHEA can greatly enhance the ability to maintain high muscle mass, but that doesn't always decrease the risk of injury. In fact, it may actually *increase* the chance of joint injury. You see, a forty-five-year-old who suddenly finds that he can bench-press 250 pounds again is very likely to forget that he is pushing that weight with middle-aged joints. And it's not just the macho men; women also notice dramatic strength improvements with DHEA and may push too far too fast. It's important to go slow when getting back in shape and to develop an awareness of connective tissue health.

YOUR CHANGING JOINTS

Your skeletal and muscle systems are designed to work together in perfect harmony, allowing your body to maintain the right mix of flexibility and rigidity. Flexibility enables us to move, dance, run, and jump. Rigidity gives control to those movements so that we don't injure ourselves. Flexibility and rigidity are regulated through the action of joints (which limit the movement of bones) along with ligaments and tendons (which hold joints together and attach muscle to bone).

As we grow older, our joints and connective tissue become parched and dried out, just like our skin. Scientists are studying an amazing group of substances known as *mucopolysaccharides*, which regulate the elasticity and resiliency of our tissues and joints. These compounds are located between the cells, where they control the level of hydration (the amount of water) available throughout our bodies, from the synovial fluid in our joints to our cartilage, ligaments, and tendons.

As we grow older, the mucopolysaccharide content of our joints and connective tissue decreases, causing a loss of resiliency and making us increasingly vulnerable to injury. What can you do to restore the structure and function of your connective tissue to youthful levels? There are two approaches to take: dietary supplementation and exercise. Both are covered in the remainder of this chapter.

SUPPLEMENTS FOR SUPPLE JOINTS

We know that mucopolysaccharides can be restored in your connective tissue through dietary supplements. The major mucopolysaccharide that keeps your joints limber is a cartilage concentrate known as *chondroitin sulfate*. Chrondroitin sulfate has been used as a therapeutic nutrient for centuries: It's a major ingredient in homemade chicken soup. At the health food store chrondroitin sulfate is usually derived from bovine cartilage. Also available are glucosamine sulfate and N-acetylglucosamine, which perform the same function.

Other important components of a connective tissue program include boron, silicon, vitamin C, magnesium, potassium, zinc, manganese, phosphorus, copper, and vitamin K. These substances, along with vitamin D and calcium, can sometimes be found in a single formulation.

WHAT ABOUT CALCIUM?

Since calcium makes up the major portion of your bone tissue, it is a vital factor in bone growth and repair. However, with all the recent hoopla over osteoporosis, we are in the midst of a calcium craze.

Just about everyone has jumped on the calcium bandwagon. Today you can wake up to a calcium-fortified glass of orange juice, pour calcium-fortified milk on your calcium-fortified breakfast cereal, and butter your toast (made with calcium-fortified flour) with calcium-fortified margarine or calcium-rich butter. Doctors are telling their patients to eat Tums®, and the limestone, dolomite, bone meal, and oyster shell business has never been better. But what good is all this calcium going to do us?

The calcium craze has two dangerous consequences. First, excessive calcium supplementation can have health risks, including impaired absorption of magnesium, iron, zinc, and possibly other minerals. Second, women who take calcium supplements for osteoporosis may ignore other, more effective approaches, such as wide-spectrum nutritional support, exercise, and hormone replacement.

THE OSTEOPOROSIS SCARE

Is osteoporosis a calcium deficiency? That's the latest misconception. Ironically, research has shown that more calcium is *not* necessarily the solution to the osteoporosis problem. Epidemiologists tell us about societies that consume less calcium than Americans do yet have a much lower incidence of osteoporosis. At the same time countries with a greater intake of calcium show no significant benefit. For example, women in the United Kingdom have an average daily intake of 990 mg of calcium in the early postmenopausal years. The average for American women is only 560 mg, yet both nations record roughly the same incidence of hip fractures.

There's no denying that osteoporosis is a tragedy. It affects over 20 million Americans every year, among whom 1.2 million people are crippled. Complications of osteoporosis kill more women than do cancers of the breast, cervix, and uterus combined. Think of it this way: Everyone hears that Aunt Tilly fell down and fractured her hip. In reality, it's more likely that Aunt Tilly's hip spontaneously fractured, causing her to fall down. Imagine living with that kind of vulnerability. In 1995 250,000 hip fractures were reported in the United States. Twenty percent of those victims never left the hospital, and 40 percent required lifelong care.

There's more. A woman can eat right, not smoke, exercise, and have a great attitude to boot, but after age thirty, she is losing minerals from her bones. She may arrive at age ninety with great muscle tone, healthy skin, a sharp mind, and plenty of organ reserves, but the structure that supports these components—her skeleton—is falling apart.

BUILDING HEALTHY BONES

Fortunately, osteoporosis is preventable, and the gradual loss of bone density can be stopped. The solution is threefold.

1. Use balanced mineral supplementation, not just calcium. Other components should include magnesium, potassium, zinc, manganese, phosphorus, boron, chromium, and copper. Vitamin C is also beneficial.

2. Get regular exercise, especially weight-bearing exercise (walking and cycling). A moderate weight-lifting routine for the upper body is also helpful, as is a regular stretching routine or yoga.

3. Establish hormone balance in your body. This is normally viewed as an estrogen issue. Hormone replacement therapy (HRT) usually includes estrogen to make up for the loss of ovarian production after menopause. However, many doctors today are including progesterone, and a growing number are looking at DHEA as an important piece of the endocrine puzzle.

DHEA AND OSTEOPOROSIS

Recent studies strongly suggest that DHEA plays an important role in maintaining bone mass as women grow older. One study of postmenopausal women found that DHEA levels were directly related to bone mineral density (BMD). In women less than sixty-nine years old there was a striking correlation between DHEA levels and the strength of their bones.

When scientists see that kind of information, they immediately wonder if there is a cause-and-effect relationship or just an association. To find out, the next step would be to give animals some DHEA and see if it strengthens their bones. They did, and it does. DHEA administration caused a significant increase in BMD in laboratory rats. What's more, researchers learned something new: DHEA can be converted to estrogen by bone cells. This in effect would produce many of the same bone-preserving benefits of estrogen replacement therapy.

We are, however, still waiting for step three, a long-term study with real live women. This needs to be done to find the dose of DHEA that will produce the greatest benefit and the least amount of risk. Since such a study, as far as I know, is not even in the planning stage, physicians are starting to experiment on their own. The benefits are simply too great to ignore.

Of course, women taking estrogen should consult with their doctor before taking DHEA supplements, as DHEA is converted to both estrogen and testosterone. Clinicians experienced in this arena are saying that DHEA may be preferable to estrogen or that we may be able to lower the amount of estrogen used in HRT. Equally intriguing are studies showing that the addition of a small amount of testosterone to estrogen replacement therapy produces improvements in energy and mood while relieving insomnia and irritability. In the future it may be possible to administer one master hormone, DHEA, instead of two or three separate hormones to get maximum results.

LET THE SUN SHINE IN

For your body to make optimum use of calcium, vitamin D is absolutely essential. The "sunshine vitamin" is manufactured by the body from the action of sunlight on bare skin. This is accomplished long before there is any reddening of the skin and requires the exposure of the face and arms to only about twenty minutes of direct sun or forty minutes of early morning or late afternoon sun. Dark-skinned

FOODS CONTAINING CALCIUM AND OTHER BONE-SUPPORT NUTRIENTS

BEANS, NUTS, AND SEEDS
Tofu
Pinto or kidney beans
Lima beans
Almonds
Sesame seeds

VEGETABLES
Broccoli
Kale
Collard greens
Green beans
Watercress
Turnip greens
Mustard greens
Okra
Parsnips
Butternut squash
Cabbage
Chinese cabbage (bok choy)
Carrots

FISH
Canned mackerel
Oysters
Herring
Salmon (with bone)
Sardines (with bone)

MILK AND MILK PRODUCTS
Low-fat milk
Yogurt, plain
Cheese

WHOLE GRAINS
Brown rice
Rolled oats
Barley flakes
Millet
Buckwheat
Whole wheat

people require about twice as long to get a day's supply of vitamin D.

Many Americans are in the habit of avoiding exposure to sunlight at all costs. We stay indoors under fluorescent lights, and when we go out, we slather sunscreen all over our bodies. This is unnatural behavior, and we are suffering for it. The sun is immune-stimulating, strengthens our bones, and enhances calcium absorption and metabolism throughout the body. Health experts now realize that our sun phobia has gone much too far. Our ancestors enjoyed full exposure to the sun for millions of years, and we can still benefit today from getting direct sun on our skin. The secret is knowing when to head for the shade. Remember, all the immune-stimulating and bone-building benefits of sunlight can be obtained before even a hint of a burn. For optimal benefit, try to get out in the sun three or four times a week.

The efficiency of your skin's natural vitamin D production diminishes with age, and this makes it important to obtain vitamin D from the diet or supplements. Vitamin D–rich foods include fatty fish, liver, eggs, and fortified milk products and breakfast cereals. Those living in northern regions as well as individuals who cannot (or choose not to) spend time outdoors should consult a physician for the proper form and amount of vitamin D supplementation.

MOVE IT, MOVE IT, MOVE IT!

Exercise is essential to the well-being of the entire skeletal system. Movement conditions and strengthens your joints and connective tissue, while inactivity deconditions the entire body, including bones, tendons, ligaments, joints, muscles, and even the nervous system.

It's important to remember that the health of bones and that of connective tissue go hand in hand. If your bones are weakening through osteoporosis, malnutrition, and lack of exercise, you can be sure that your connective tissue is deteriorating as well. Bones and muscles work together, and strong muscles can relieve much of the strain on bones. In addition, developing your muscles actually strengthens the underlying bones. Studies show, for example, that the bone density of the lower spine is directly proportionate to the strength of the lower back muscles.

Your exercise program need not be strenuous, but it must be consistent. If you are elderly or have special needs, a physician, certified personal trainer, or physical therapist can assist you in setting up an individualized exercise program. Weight-bearing exercises such as walking or cycling are excellent and provide movement that is less jarring than jogging or jumping rope. Moderate weight lifting will also do much to strengthen the muscles and bones of the upper body. Although swimming is a great form of exercise, it is not weight-bearing, and so it will not be as helpful in your program of connective tissue strengthening.

Ideally, exercise should begin in childhood and continue throughout life. Research shows that even elderly and "fragile" individuals can benefit greatly from carefully designed exercise programs.

ACHIEVING FULL RANGE OF MOTION

When we were in the primordial forests, we moved constantly. Our bodies experienced a full range of motion without us having to think about it. In the twentieth century we have to make an extra effort to obtain full range of motion when we exercise. Most of us tend to repeat the same movements over and over, and that strengthens our joints only in one direction.

For example, if your knees only flex and extend, you're not working the tendons and ligaments on either side of the knee. And if those ligaments are deconditioned, you'll be more prone to injury. Our knee, elbow, and shoulder joints deserve special attention when we exercise. To get the full range of motion you need to add a form of flexibility training such as yoga or a comprehensive stretching routine that challenges the ligaments and tendons along a number of planes.

COUCH POTATOES: AN ENDANGERED SPECIES

Think about this. In our species, as in every other species on the planet, those individuals with the best survival skills survive and reproduce, passing on their skills to the next generation. If you were in charge, what would you do with an organism that just sat there?

That's right: You'd eliminate it. You'd insert DNA cues that would activate self-destruct mechanisms through various tissues and organs to hasten its exit from the planet. That way there would be room for more highly motivated, active organisms to thrive and ensure the survival of the species.

If you want to maintain high-level wellness, your first and foremost goal should be to send a message to your cells every day that *this is an active body*. I don't mean to scare you, but I'll do whatever it takes to get you off the couch! The next chapter will give you more information on developing the exercise component of your DHEA Plan.

BIBLIOGRAPHY

Altura BM, Altura BT, et al. Magnesium deficiency and hypertension: Correlation between magnesium-deficient diets and microcirculatory changes in situ. *Science* 1984; 223:1315–7.

Altura BT, Brust M, Bloom S, et al. Magnesium dietary intake modulates blood lipid levels and atherogenesis. *Proc Natl Acad Sci USA* 1990; 87:1840–4.

Anderson RA, et al. Chromium intake, absorption and excretion of subjects consuming self-selected diets. *Am J Clin Nutr* 1985; 41:1177–83.

Anderson RA, Polansky MM, et al. Effect of chromium supplementation on insulin, insulin binding and C-peptide values of hypoglycemic human subjects. *Am J Clin Nutr* 1985; 41:841–8.

Anderson RA. Nutritional role of chromium. *Sci Total Environ* 1981; 17:13–29.

Atik OS. Zinc and senile osteoporosis. *J Am Geriatr Soc* 1983; 31:790.

Bhambhani MM, Bates CJ, Crisp AJ. Plasma ascorbic acid concentrations in osteoporotic outpatients. *B J Rheumatol* 1992; 31(2):142–3.

Bjorntorp P. Exercise in the treatment of obesity. *Clin Endocrinol Metab* 1976; 5:431–7.

Campbell WW, Polansky MM, et al. Exercise training and dietary chromium effects on glycogen, glycogen synthase, phosporylase and total protein in rats. *J Nutr* 1989; 119:653–60.

Carlisle EM. Silicon: a requirement in bone formation independent of vitamin D1. *Calcif Tissue Int* 1981; 33(1):27–34.

Chesnut CH III. Is osteoporosis a pediatric disease? Peak bone mass attainment in the adolescent female. *Public Health Rep* 1989; 104 (Suppl):50.

Conte A, Palmieri L, Segnini D, Ronca G. Metabolic fate of partially depolymerized chondroitin sulfate administered to the rat. *Drugs Exp Clin Res* 1991; 17(1):27–33.

Dawson-Hughes B, Dallal GE, Krall EA, Sadowski L, Sahyoun N, Tannenbaum S. A controlled trial of the effect of calcium supplementation on bone density in postmenopausal women. *N Eng J Med*, 1990; 323(13):878–83.

Deehr MS, Dallal GE, Smith KT, Taulbee JD, Dawson-Hughes B. Effects of different calcium sources on iron absorption in postmenopausal women. *Am J Clin Nutr* 1990; 51(1):95–9.

DeFronzo RA. Obesity is associated with impaired insulin-mediated potassium uptake. *Metabolism* 1988; 2:105–8.

Felig P. Hypothesis: Insulin is the mediator of feeding-related thermogenesis: Insulin resistance and/or deficiency results in a thermogenic defect which contributes to the pathogenesis of obesity. *Clin Physiol* 1984; 4:267–76.

Folkers K, Wolaniuk A. Research on Coenzyme Q10 in clinical medicine and in immunomodulation. *Drugs Exp Clin Res* 1985; XI(8):539–45.

Franceschi RT, Young J. Regulation of alkaline phosphatase by 1,25-dihydroxy-vitamin D3 and ascorbic acid in bone-derived cells. *J Bone Mineral Res* 1990; 5(11):1157.

Hardingham T, Bayliss M. Proteoglycans of articular cartilage: Changes in aging and in joint disease. *Semin Arthritis Rheum* 1990; 20(3 Suppl 1):12–33.

Hart JP, Shearer MJ, et al. Electrochemical detection of depressed circulating levels of vitamin K in osteoporosis. *J Clin Endocrinol Metab* 1985; 60:1268–9.

Hicks JT. Treatment of fatigue in general practice: A double blind study. *Clin Med* 1964; 71:85–90.

Holt PR, Rosenberg IH, Russell RM. Causes and consequences of hypochlorhydria in the elderly. *Dig Dis Sci* 1989; 34(6):933.

Kahn A, Pottenger LA, Phillips FM, Viola RW. Evidence of proteoglycan/proteoglycan interactions within aggregates. *J Orthop Res* 1991; 9(6):777–86.

Kamei M, Fujita T, et al. The distribution and content of ubiquinone (coenzyme Q) in foods. *Int J Vitam Nutr Res* 1986; 56:57–65.

Langsjoen PH, Folkers K, Lyson K, Muratsu K, Lyson T, Langsjoen P. Effective and safe therapy with Coenzyme Q10 for cardiomyopathy. *Klin Wochenschr* 1988; 66:583–90.

Lenay G (ed.). *Coenzyme Q: Biochemistry, Bioenergetics and Clinical Applications of Ubiquinone.* Wiley, New York, 1985.

Luyten FP, Verbruggen G, Veys EM, Goffin E, De Pypere H. In vitro repair potential of articular cartilage: Proteoglycan metabolism in the different areas of the femoral condyles in human cartilage explants. *J Rheumatol* 1987; 14(2):329–34.

Marconi C, Sassi G, Cerretelli P. The effect of an alpha ketoglutarate-pyridoxine complex on human maximal aerobic and anaerobic performance. *Eur J Appl Physiol* 1982; 49:307–17.

Miller DD. Calcium in the diet: Food sources, recommended intakes, and nutritional bioavailability. *Adv Food Nutri Res* 1989; 33:103.

Mills CF, Bremner I, Chesters JK (eds.). *Trace Elements in Man and Animals,* Vol 5. Commonwealth Agricultural Bureau, London, 1984.

Morgan KJ, Stampley GL. Dietary intake levels and food sources of magnesium and calcium for selected segments of the US population. *Magnesium* 1988; 7(5–6):225–33.

Nawata H, Tanaka S, Takayanagi R, et al. Aromatase in bone cell: Association with osteoporosis in postmenopausal women. *J Steroid Biochem Molec Biol* 1995; 53(1–6):165–74.

Palmieri L, Conte A, Giovannini L, Lualdi P, Ronca G. Metabolic fate of exogenous chondroitin sulfate in the experimental animal. *Arzneimittelforschung* 1990; 40(3):319–23.

Recker RR. Low bone mass may not be the only cause of skeletal fragility in osteoporosis. *Proc Soc Exp Biol Med* 1989; 191(3):272–4.

Riis B, Thomsen K, Christiannsen C. Does calcium supplementation prevent postmenopausal bone loss? *N Engl J Med* 1987; 316:173.

Rude RK, Adams JS, et al. Low serum concentrations of 1,25-dihydroxyvitamin D in human magnesium deficiency. *J Clin Endocrinol Metab* 1985; 61:933.

Schwarz K. A bound form of silicon in glycosaminoglycans and polyuronides. *Proc Natl Acad Sci USA* 1973; 70:1608.

Shils ME. Magnesium, calcium and parathyroid hormone interactions. *Ann NY Acad Sci* 1980; 355:165.

Uotila L. The metabolic functions and mechanism of action of vitamin K. *Scand J Clin Lab Investi Suppl* 1990; 201:109–17.

Van Gaal L, De Leeuw, et al. Exploratory study of coenzyme Q10 in obesity. *Biomedical and Clinical Aspects of Coenzyme Q*, Vol 4. K Folkers and Y Yamamura (eds.). Elsevier, New York, 1984, 369–73.

Waddell TG, Henderson BS, Morris RT, Lewis CM, Zimmermann AG. Chemical evolution of the citric acid cycle: Sunlight photolysis of alphaketoglutaric acid. *Orig Life Evol Biosph* 1987; 17(2):149–53.

Yamaguchi M, Sakashita T. Enhancement of vitamin D3 effect on bone metabolism in weanling rats orally administered zinc sulfate. *Acta Endocrinol* 1986; 111:285.

CHAPTER 7

DHEA and Exercise

For the past twenty-five years we've been hearing from health professionals, fitness gurus, and the media about the benefits of regular exercise. We've seen an incredible boom in the fitness industry: health clubs, home exercise equipment, workout clothes, high-priced "training" shoes, and a multitude of video workouts brought to us by stunning bodies.

In spite of this fitness "boom," the average American is less fit than ever. Today 60 percent of American adults are completely sedentary, which means they get no regular exercise at all. If you think of the exercise craze as a parade, most people are on the sidelines watching it go by. The parade participants were fit to start with, and they are even more fit when they finish.

To attract people to their products, the fitness industry once showcased the most beautiful and fit individuals. However, when we subscribed to the magazines, bought the Exercycles, signed up for the health clubs, and watched the videos, we found one major problem: It was easier to fail than it was to succeed.

The truth is that only a small percentage of the nation got excited and motivated, bought the stuff, and "just did it." A much larger percentage bought the stuff, tried it for a while, and then consigned it to a corner of the garage; the largest percentage of all did nothing. In reality, the exercise "boom" was a bust. The latest Surgeon General's report (July 1995) confirms that physical activity is extremely important to your health, but no one seems to know how to get Americans moving.

DHEA MAKES EXERCISE EASIER

Most people assume that American adults don't exercise because they don't have time or are too busy. I disagree. As evidence, I can point to any gym or health club. Invariably, the busiest people in town are working out. Exercise makes them even more productive, because *exercise produces energy.*

The good news is that the DHEA Plan sets the stage for you to enjoy and benefit from exercise like never before. Why? Because it will increase your metabolic efficiency and enhance your body's production of energy. When you have abundant energy, no one has to make you feel guilty or beg you to exercise; it comes naturally. If you're also strengthening your bones and connective tissue (see Chapter 6), you'll be ready to experience what I call high-level fitness. Even if the fitness parade passed you by, you now have a chance to catch up. The DHEA Plan is a way for *everyone* to participate.

EXERCISE AND EVOLUTION

A woman complained to her doctor, "My husband just sits on the couch all day, drinking beer and eating potato chips and watching TV." The doctor replied, "Oh, that won't last long." The woman was surprised. "You mean he's going to snap out of that lifestyle?" The doctor responded, "Well, he might, but what I was referring to is that *he* won't last long. He'll be dead."

The truth is, a sedentary life is a short life—thanks to our Paleolithic programming. Needless to say, our Paleolithic ancestors were able to maintain optimum fitness levels without ever setting foot in a health club. In fact, the training we do in health clubs today is a way of duplicating the strength-building activities our ancestors did naturally for 1.6 million years. Think of it as a way to get back in sync with your genes.

Like most modern adults, you already know that exercise will make you feel better, look better, and live longer, but you're too tired to even begin. And then, from lack of exercise, you gain weight. It's a vicious cycle, but it can be broken.

You'll never know how good you can feel until you experience high-level fitness. The remainder of this chapter provides an outline of how to get there from wherever you may be and how DHEA can help.

EXERCISE AND AGING

Your doctor will tell you dozens of benefits you can get from exercise, and all of it is true. The problem is that our metabolism changes as we age, and as a result, we don't respond to exercise the way we used to. Instead of being invigorating, exercise becomes a chore or, worse, an opportunity for injury.

As we grow older, performing the same amounts and types of exercise we did in our youth may be interpreted by the body as stress. This increases the production of the stress hormone cortisol, which will actually lower DHEA, suppress immunity, and contribute to a number of degenerative problems.

Exercise naturally produces what is known as a *catabolic* (breakdown) phase. Catabolism is the breaking down of energy stores and proteins in the body, and this is a normal stage of exercise. A young person quickly shifts from the catabolic to the *anabolic* (building up) phase as soon as the exercise period is over. Proteins are then quickly resynthesized, and this is important for the maintenance of lean muscle.

When you are older and your cortisol level increases with exercise, it keeps the body in the catabolic phase. That means your recovery from a workout is delayed. Even more significant, protein repair and resynthesis are delayed or incomplete, resulting in gradual loss of muscle mass. DHEA can change that.

DHEA BUILDS ENERGY AND MUSCLE MASS

DHEA can decrease your recovery time after a workout and dramatically improve muscle repair and synthesis. This stems from the ability of DHEA to raise levels of the repair biochemical IGF-1. Gerontologists have known for decades that IGF-1 decreases as we age, and they used to consider it part and parcel of the aging process. "Oh, well, the body gets old. It can't repair proteins. It falls apart and dies. That's life." Now scientists are wondering if this type of decline is really inevitable.

Recently, a team of researchers gave 100 mg of DHEA to a group of men in their late fifties. After only thirty days they documented an astounding 90 percent increase in IGF-1. This translates into greater muscle gains for athletes over thirty, better muscle maintenance for anyone over fifty, and, just as important as these anabolic benefits, decreased risk for heart disease. IGF-1 stimulates the production of nitric oxide (NO), which dilates blood vessels, improves circulation, and helps prevent the formation of abnormal clots.

Another benefit people taking DHEA often notice is a marked improvement in muscle definition as soon as they start strength training. An excellent study in the *Annals of the New York Academy of Sciences* concluded:

> DHEA in appropriate replacement doses appears to have remedial effects with respect to its ability to induce an anabolic growth factor, increase muscle strength and lean body mass, activate immune function, and enhance quality of life in aging men and women, with no significant adverse effects.[1]

Keeping DHEA levels at prime peak is extremely important for anyone wishing to stay active into the eighties, nineties, and beyond. When you combine this with optimum levels of bioenergetic nutrients and a bone-building and joint-protecting program (see Chapter 8), you'll see a rapid improvement in your energy level as well as maximum benefits from regular exercise. This is the way to get motivated, not by beating yourself up with "shoulds" and "oughts."

THE CRITICAL HURDLE: ADAPTATION

The unfit people who tried to join the exercise parade found themselves experiencing sore muscles, blistered feet, exhaustion, and often

GUIDELINES FOR PEAK FITNESS

Here's a summary of what you can do to ensure optimum levels of fitness for decades to come:

1. Monitor your DHEA levels to maintain prime peak.
2. Use DHEA supplements if needed.
3. Do not overexercise. You should feel invigorated after your workout, not exhausted or depressed.
4. Use bioenergetics to enhance your metabolic efficiency.
5. Use a connective tissue support program to protect your joints, tendons, ligaments, and bones from injury.

depression. They began to make excuses: not enough time, too many other things to do, too far to drive, too cold, too hot, I don't want to mess up my hair.

What they meant was "I don't like all this pain and exhaustion. This isn't making me feel better; it's making me feel worse." Few programs are designed to assure success for people who are just beginning an exercise routine. And, most people aren't told about the four- to six-week adaptation period it takes for their bodies to adjust to the new exercise routines.

Adaptation is the stage between the unfit state and the fit state. It's a metabolic no-man's-land where you are making increased energy demands on your body but your body doesn't yet know where or how to obtain the energy. Few people make it through this stage because, while in it, they often feel like they've been hit by a bus. Instead of feeling invigorated by exercise, they feel wiped out. Instead of the natural appetite suppression that fit people experience after a workout, they often feel ravenous hunger and a craving for sweets. And it hurts—physically and emotionally. It's very demoralizing to be exhausted to the point of fainting while the aerobics instructor or fitness guru is hardly breaking a sweat.

It's no wonder that for every ten people who start workout

programs, six drop out in the first month. The tragedy is, if you've tried time and again to start an exercise program without success, you've probably never felt the intense joy of being invigorated by exercise. That's not your fault. The metabolic "deck" has been stacked against you. The good news is that the DHEA Plan can change all that forever.

A DOZEN BENEFITS OF EXERCISE

1. **EXERCISE BURNS CALORIES.** Combined with reduced caloric intake and improved metabolic efficiency, exercise is the key to long-term weight management.

2. **EXERCISE USES FAT AS FUEL.** For about the first thirty minutes of exercise the body uses blood glucose, glycogen (stored glucose), and a little fat. After thirty minutes the body burns mostly fat.

3. **EXERCISE INCREASES MUSCLE MASS.** This is perhaps the most important benefit of exercise because increased muscle mass has profound effects on metabolism, bone strength, and weight management throughout life. A pound of muscle will typically burn from one hundred to four hundred times the number of calories burned by a pound of fat. Someone with a high muscle mass therefore can consume more calories without gaining weight. Remember, muscle mass refers not to bodybuilder muscles but to the overall percentage of nonfat tissue on your body. You can increase your muscle mass considerably without ever looking like a bodybuilder.

DHEA is the key because after age forty it becomes difficult for women and even men to increase muscle mass. It's as if nature were saying, "Why bother? This organism is over the hill." DHEA can literally move the hill by stimulating production of IGF-1, your body's muscle-building, tissue-repairing youth biochemical. And there does not seem to be an age at which this benefit disappears. Studies with men and women have documented significant IGF-1 stimulation in every age group tested.

4. **EXERCISE DECREASES APPETITE.** Metabolic suppression of appetite is a result of fitness that takes time to achieve. Studies show, however, that moderate-intensity exercise can also decrease appetite by affecting the hypothalamus, the brain's appetite control center. This

effect on the hypothalamus occurs even before the body reaches a high level of fitness. Importantly, DHEA may also be a factor here. In animal studies DHEA administration leads to decreased food consumption and weight loss, resulting apparently from an increase in the level of serotonin in the hypothalamus. Coincidentally, this is one of the properties of fenfluramine, a drug recently approved for weight loss.

5. EXERCISE HELPS REDUCE STRESS AND DEPRESSION, COMMON CAUSES OF OVEREATING. Studies show that moderate exercise stimulates the production of "feel-good" hormones called *endorphins* and pain-relieving hormones called *enkephalins*. These hormones, combined with the natural exuberance that comes with being active, lead to more successful stress management and mood elevation. As was described in Chapter 4, that causes the body to produce more DHEA, putting you into an exciting upward spiral. Feeling good relieves stress, successful stress management increases DHEA, increased DHEA gives you more positive results from exercise, better results lead to higher motivation, which makes you feel even better, and so on.

6. EXERCISE REDUCES THE RISK OF HEART DISEASE, AMERICA'S NUMBER-ONE KILLER. Exercise lowers blood pressure, increases the levels of "good" high-density lipoprotein (HDL) cholesterol in the blood while decreasing "bad" LDL and very low density lipoprotein (VLDL) cholesterol levels, decreases blood triglycerides, and strengthens the heart muscle. Studies also show that exercise helps people quit smoking, which is a major contributor to heart disease.

7. EXERCISE HELPS CONTROL DIABETES. Blood sugar is in part regulated by exercise and diet. Studies show that with weight loss and exercise, nearly 50 percent of adult-onset diabetic patients are able to discontinue insulin and diabetic drug use. There is even evidence that exercise can help prevent diabetes in those with a genetic predisposition for this devastating disease.

8. EXERCISE PROMOTES DEEPER, MORE RESTFUL SLEEP. However, exercising right before going to bed can make it more difficult to fall asleep.

9. RHYTHMIC EXERCISE RELIEVES CONSTIPATION. Walking, running, swimming, cycling, and rowing all promote bowel regularity. Walking has the added benefit of enhancing the digestion and metabolism of food.

10. EXERCISE STIMULATES THE LYMPHATIC SYSTEM. This system is the body's "garbage disposal" for metabolic debris, dead cells, and recycled waste. Improving lymphatic circulation can contribute significantly to overall health.

11. RANGE-OF-MOTION EXERCISE IMPROVES FLEXIBILITY AND STRENGTH. Range-of-motion exercises such as yoga and stretching are especially important. These exercises increase the fluid that lubricates joints, improve the flexibility and strength of connective tissue, and can have profound effects on a wide range of degenerative disorders, including rheumatoid arthritis, osteoarthritis, bursitis, and tendinitis.

12. EXERCISE LEADS TO FEELINGS OF STRENGTH AND IMPROVED SELF-ESTEEM. Feeling strong enhances self-esteem and provides a feeling of being capable and in control. These feelings can have profound effects in many areas of life for both men and women. Self-esteem is very much a subconscious thing. Positive thinking is all well and good, but if there is an old tape playing in your subconscious telling you that you're a wimp, all the affirmations in the world won't improve your feeling of self-worth. That tape might have been placed there decades ago by a parent or other authority figure, but it's still influencing the way you feel about yourself.

Exercise and the resulting strength benefits can banish such deep feelings of lack and limitation. Why is that? Evolution. For over a million years the most important skills were all related to strength. Your genes know nothing about other attributes you may possess, such as the ability to manage a stock portfolio and amass a fortune. That may gain for you the approval of others and please your conscious mind, but your subconscious wants to know if you can wrestle a bear and win. Think about that the next time you're in a health club. The men and women you see lifting weights are not pushing that intense activity just to look good. They are, knowingly or unknowingly, satisfying a deep inner need for self-esteem in the form of physical strength.

THE WEEKEND WARRIOR SYNDROME

Are you a "weekend warrior"? Do you devote five days a week to sedentary living, followed by a Saturday or Sunday of strenuous exercise? If so, you're probably experiencing more pain than gain. You'll get the most benefit from exercise if it's spread out over the entire week rather than concentrated in a day or two. You don't need to become a weekend warrior seven days a week; on the contrary, slow and steady wins the fitness race. It's not about "buns of steel" or Terminator biceps. If you're just starting out with exercise, follow these principles.

EXERCISE SHOULD BE MODERATE. Fatigue and exhaustion can slow your progress toward fitness and weight loss. Moderate exercise stimulates your metabolic systems without throwing your body into "adaptation." Avoid the "no pain, no gain" mentality at all costs.

CONSISTENCY IS MORE IMPORTANT THAN INTENSITY. There's a "warehouse manager" in your brain that predicts your energy needs on the basis of past experience. If you lead a sedentary life, the warehouse manager knows that little energy is needed and most excess calories are sent into storage (on your thighs, for example). Sporadic exercise only confuses the manager. One day the manager runs out of energy, and the next day there's a surplus. The net result is that your body experiences no real increase in metabolic efficiency or fat burning.

However, when you do consistent, moderate exercise, the message to your brain is this: "This body is now an active, dynamic body that requires a great deal more energy than before, so I need to stop storing so many calories as fat and keep more in ready reserve for all this activity." The good news is that to make this message loud and clear, the exercise doesn't have to be intense or even long. The most important thing is consistency.

USE THE ACTIVITY BREAK CONCEPT. When you first add exercise to your daily routine, you want to send as many "activity messages" as possible to the energy warehouse manager in your brain. You want the manager to know that your active body is going to require increasing levels of energy.

Studies show that an activity such as gardening, housework, golf, bowling, shopping, or badminton can contribute to improved fitness and greater metabolic efficiency, so get in the habit of taking an "activity break" every couple of hours. Each activity break should be at least ten minutes long.

In fact, it is best not to sit for more than two hours at a time at work or at home. Keep the messages going to the brain that your body is in motion and needs energy. Not only do activity breaks stimulate

your metabolism, but research shows that they also enhance productivity and decrease days lost to illness.

Here's a brief list of activity breaks that can effectively send the
right message to your brain's warehouse manager:

- Walk your dog.
- Dance or move rhythmically to music for ten minutes.
- Walk around the parking lot or to another department in your
  company.
- Stretch or do some gentle yoga or tai chi movements.
- Spend ten minutes on an Exercycle or treadmill.
- Clean the house.
- Skip rope gently.
- Find a hula-hoop and learn how to keep it going.
- Juggle.
- Throw a Frisbee.
- Jump on a mini-trampoline.
- Do an exercise routine with hand weights.
- Roller-skate.
- Swing.
- Wash your car.

DURATION IS CRITICAL IF FAT BURNING IS YOUR GOAL. It takes about thirty
minutes for your metabolism to switch from burning primarily carbohydrates to burning mostly fat. Every minute you exercise beyond the
thirty-minute threshold is a fat-burning minute.

DHEA AND BIOENERGETIC SUPPLEMENTS HELP MINIMIZE ADAPTATION. DHEA
and the bioenergetic nutrients discussed in Chapter 6 mobilize your
metabolism, providing the energy needed to support the increased
activity level of your body. Increasing exercise without these important tools is like trying to run your car with a spark plug missing.
You'll move, but your efforts will lack power and the results will be
disappointing. Optimizing bioenergetic nutrient levels and keeping
DHEA at prime peak will help you blaze through adaptation and
experience an entirely new level of energy and vitality.

Note: When your muscles work, they produce by-products of
energy metabolism known as free radicals. Normally, free radicals are
neutralized by other biochemicals in your body known as antioxi-

dants. But by increasing the metabolic efficiency and work capacity of your muscles, DHEA may cause an increase in free radical production. Animal studies show that this can be completely offset by increasing your intake of antioxidants, especially vitamin E. See Chapter 9 for specific supplement recommendations.

YOUR DHEA EXERCISE PROGRAM

The following is a sample exercise program that can take you all the way from the very beginning level to the most advanced level of fitness. Be prepared to devote six to twelve weeks to each step (steps one and two can take place simultaneously).

STEP ONE: Get a metabolic "tune-up." Find out your DHEA level and supplement it if necessary to reach prime peak (see Chapter 11). Start taking bioenergetic nutrients on a daily basis (see Chapter 6).

STEP TWO: Get active by taking frequent activity breaks.

STEP THREE: Establish a fitness base through walking. Start with twenty minutes of walking three times a week and work up to thirty minutes of walking five times a week.

STEP FOUR: Build fat-burning minutes; three or four times a week will add extra minutes to your walking base. Gradually work up to an extra thirty to sixty minutes per walk.

STEP FIVE: After six weeks of walking, enlist the help of a certified fitness trainer and add twenty minutes of strength training with weights twice a week. Gradually work up to strength training every other day.

STEP SIX: With the help of your fitness trainer, continue increasing the intensity of your workouts until you reach your maximal workout level.

STEP SEVEN: Stretch daily throughout your entire exercise program, from the beginning to the advanced level.

THE FIT PRINCIPLE

The initials FIT stand for *frequency, intensity,* and *time,* and you adjust these three factors as your exercise program progresses. You can start exercising twice a week and then increase the *frequency* of your workouts; you can then increase their *intensity* (walking up hills instead of on flat terrain or jogging instead of walking); finally, you can increase the *time or duration* of each exercise session.

Use the FIT formula to customize your exercise program for maximum comfort, enjoyment, and benefits. Now, let's begin.

THE UNIVERSAL EXERCISE: WALKING

For a beginning exercise routine to be effective, it must meet four criteria:

- Enjoyable—no one will do something he or she dislikes for very long.
- Easy to do—something everyone can do without lessons or training.
- Inexpensive—no expensive equipment, memberships, or special clothing required.
- Efficient—gives people the most benefit for the amount of time spent.

You already know which form of exercise meets all these criteria: *walking.* Walking is popular because it's an activity almost anyone can do. It doesn't require special ability or athletic skill and can be done almost anywhere at almost any time. It is incredibly efficient because it utilizes the largest muscles of your body—the front and back of your thighs.

Walking can be done in your home or neighborhood, on wilderness trails, at the beach, or at the local shopping mall. It is easy to do, yields enormous benefits, and seldom causes injury or discomfort. However, there are a few guidelines to be aware of.

FORGET ABOUT "TARGET PULSE" AND HEART RATE. If you are at high risk for heart disease or are recovering from heart surgery, target pulse can be very important. For the rest of us, walking at a steady rate that allows us to breathe comfortably but doesn't allow moss to grow under our feet will bring us the benefits of exercise. Don't worry about walking at a "brisk pace" in the beginning; just get out and walk. "Brisk" will come when you're ready. One maxim to remember: If you're moving, you're exercising.

DON'T OVEREXERT YOURSELF. Here's an easy way to make sure you're not overdoing it: Watch your breathing. If you can walk and talk without gasping, you're okay. At that pace your muscles are getting the oxygen they need to burn fat. If you start huffing and puffing or can't carry on a conversation, that means you are in oxygen debt. This is not only potentially dangerous, it's inefficient. If your muscles can't get the oxygen they need to burn fat, they'll burn glucose or protein from muscle tissue. In other words, exercise that is too high in intensity for your level of fitness can cause you to lose muscle mass—the very thing you're trying to build up.

DURATION. Remember that after thirty minutes of walking, every minute is a fat-burning minute that adds to your fitness level. At that point you are forcing your body to use fat as fuel. When this activity is repeated regularly, the warehouse manager in your brain will instruct your body to produce more fat-burning enzymes and other biochemicals that will provide more energy. The longer you walk, the greater the benefit . . . as long as you don't get blisters or exhaust yourself.

STAY COOL. Overweight individuals commonly have a reduced ability to dissipate body heat owing to the extra "insulation" they carry around. For this reason some may find it more comfortable to schedule walking time in the morning or evening hours. Air-conditioned shopping malls are great walking sites, especially when the humidity is high. Avoid stretchy synthetic "workout" wear and go with comfortable, loose-fitting, natural fiber clothing.

EQUIPMENT. Good walking shoes are highly recommended and should be worn with high-quality cotton-blend athletic socks. Look for comfort and support, avoiding shoes that rub your heels or pinch your toes.

FOOT CARE. If your feet hurt or get blistered, that will stop your walking program cold. Be on the lookout for blisters. Keep your feet clean and dry; light absorbent powder or baking soda can help remove perspiration. Keep your toenails trimmed in a straight line to prevent injuries.

BE FLEXIBLE. Don't limit yourself to scheduled walking times. Take advantage of every opportunity. Walk to the store, the bank, or the park with your kids. Park a few blocks away from the office or walk up the stairs instead of taking the elevator. Every step counts.

WARM UP. While it's not necessary to stretch your legs and ankles as you see runners doing, it's a good idea to begin your walk at a slow pace. This natural "warm-up" prevents injury and pain and gives your body a chance to ease into a full-paced walking stride. (Feel free to stretch if you want, however. It feels wonderful and is a great way to loosen tight joints and muscles. Just make sure it's gentle stretching with no bouncing, overextension, or pain.)

POSTURE. During your walk, stop once or twice and check your posture. Shrug your shoulders tightly for ten or fifteen seconds to relieve any stress in the upper back and raise one knee at a time as high as you can to loosen the hips. As you walk, you can avoid neck pain by looking ahead rather than down. Try to have the shoulders comfortably back and be sure to swing your arms briskly in time with your legs.

COOL DOWN. Slow down for the last two or three minutes of your walk. After you finish, do a few knee raises to relieve lower back stress. A nice, slow "rag doll" forward bend from the waist (with the knees slightly bent) will help you relax and stretch the muscles you just used.

WEATHERPROOF YOUR SCHEDULE. Don't let bad weather stop your progress. Develop your exercise options in advance so you don't have to worry about what to do when the blizzard hits or the temperature zooms to 110. Some popular options are walking in the mall, working out at the YMCA or health club, and using a home Exercycle or treadmill while watching television or reading.

YOUR FITNESS BASE

To establish a level of fitness that will help you feel better, have more energy, and achieve your weight management goals, you need to walk at least thirty minutes a day five times per week. Of course, you don't have to start out at that level. Instead, start with a time and pace that are comfortable for you and work up gradually. If you start out slowly, you will feel good and want to walk farther as your level of fitness increases.

If you're feeling good, don't limit yourself to five days a week. Walking every day is fine, but walking less than five times a week lets your warehouse manager forget that yours is an active body that needs more energy. Commitment to a consistent walking program is an essential first step.

In the beginning you may need to pay special attention to your motivation and do everything possible to make walking enjoyable. Find pleasant places to walk so you can enjoy the beauty that surrounds you and think about the wonderful things going on in your body. Feel yourself getting more fit, more energetic, and more in control of your life.

To get the benefit of fat burning, add long-duration exercise to your base. Try to have three or four sessions per week in which you walk for sixty or even ninety minutes.

Had enough of walking? Now that your overall fitness quotient is up, try varying your routine. Aerobics classes, bicycling, tennis, and any other sport that gets your heart pumping are great.

THE NEXT LEVEL: STRENGTH TRAINING

To maximize the benefit of all the exercise you're getting, you need to increase your upper body strength. Sixty-five percent of your muscles are above the waist, and these may be your most underdeveloped muscles.

Exercises such as walking, jogging, tennis, basketball, and racquetball emphasize the major muscle groups in the legs and provide relatively little benefit to the upper body muscles. The easiest place to build muscle mass quickly is in the upper body. Remember, we're not talking about the pumping-iron muscles. We're talking about building muscle tissue and tone. Research shows that using light weights (3 to 5 pounds to start) can effectively and efficiently strengthen muscles.

GETTING STARTED

You may want to join a health club or use the services of a certified fitness trainer to help you develop an exercise routine to strengthen your upper body. There are two major advantages to using fitness trainers: They can help you learn to perform each exercise safely and correctly, and they can provide advice about when to increase weight or repetitions. Just be sure that any fitness trainer you use is properly certified; a trainer without credentials can be hazardous to your health.

If a fitness trainer is not available, you can use the following routine, which I have found to be very safe and helpful. Try to do twenty minutes at least twice a week, building up to four times a week. Most men and women can begin this series with 3-pound hand weights. When repeating an exercise fifteen times becomes easy, increase the weight for that exercise. I recommend increasing in 1-pound increments to avoid injury. Ultimately, you may be performing some of these exercises with weights of 10 pounds or more. Just remember to go slowly.

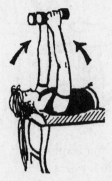

BENCH FLY. Lie on a bench and hold weights straight up over your chest with elbows slightly bent. Holding the same bend in your elbows, slowly lower your arms outward in a semicircular arc until the weights are level with your chest or slightly lower. Bring the weights back up over your chest. Repeat five times and work up to fifteen times.

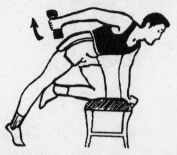

TRICEPS EXTENSION. Support the left knee and left hand on a bench or chair. Hold the weight in the right hand at the side of your chest, keeping your arm bent so that your elbow is behind you. Without moving the elbow, extend your arm behind you. Bring your arm back to the starting position. Repeat five times and work up to fifteen. Repeat with the left arm.

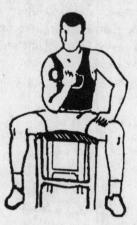

CURLS. Sit leaning forward with your legs slightly spread and the left hand on the left thigh. Keeping the right elbow on the right thigh, hold a weight so that your forearm is horizontal. Slowly curl the weight up and in toward your chest; lower and repeat five times and then work up to fifteen. Repeat with the left arm.

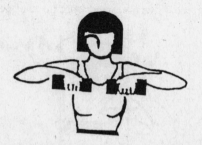

UPRIGHT ROW. Stand with your feet shoulder width apart with the knees unlocked and hold the weights side by side (palms toward thighs). Slowly pull them up to your collarbone until your elbows are just above shoulder height. Slowly lower and repeat five times; work up to fifteen times.

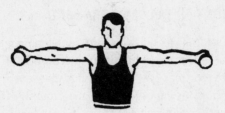

LATERAL RAISE. Stand with your feet shoulder width apart and your knees unlocked. Hold the weights at your sides at thigh level. Slowly lift the weights out to the sides to shoulder level, keeping the elbows slightly bent. Slowly lower and repeat five times; then work up to fifteen times.

The important thing to remember is that these exercises should be slow and controlled. Never jerk the weights or overextend your joints.

Do all five exercises slowly, concentrating on the movement of each muscle group. Feel how your muscles move and notice which ones seem to be stronger or weaker. After you complete the exercises, you can repeat the entire set until you have filled your twenty minutes.

Important Note: Strength training should be done *every other day* so that your muscles have time to rest and build between training sessions. You must stick with your strength training program for six to twelve weeks at a time to see results. Then move on to the next challenge.

WHAT ABOUT EXERCISE VIDEOS?

Exercise videos can be a real boon if no fitness trainers are available in your area. Although there are at least two dozen muscle-building videos on the market, most are of poor quality and some are dangerous. After reviewing all the top videos, the three I would recommend are *Keys to Weight Training, Volume One* with Bill Pearl (KTWT

Productions, Ltd.), the *Weight Watchers Series* on upper body toning (Time-Life Video), and *Working Out with Weights* with Jane Fonda.

THE FINAL FRONTIER: MAXIMAL TRAINING

The term *maximal training* refers to a strength training program that works your muscles *to the max*. In this advanced workout, for example, you may do just ten "reps" per exercise, but you use so much weight that the eleventh rep is impossible. Maximal training is the most efficient use of your time and energy, but you need to build up to it slowly and under the supervision of a qualified fitness trainer. In addition, if you are over forty, be sure to utilize the joint, bone, and tendon support nutrients described in Chapter 6.

Men tend to get into maximal training more than women do because of sheer testosterone. You can see it in the machine and free weight area of any gym. All the guys are groaning like primates because that's what it takes to maximize a muscle's capability. Ask the fellow who's just finished a 250-pound bench press how he feels. He's had to gather every ounce of strength in his shoulders, arms, chest, and back to do it, and he feels *fantastic*. His self-esteem shoots up; there is literally no difference between him and the gorilla who's head of the pack. Like the gorilla, he's simply acting out his DNA instructions.

Women have not historically done maximal weight training for two reasons. First, they didn't know they could or weren't given the option. Second, most women have an aversion to "bulking up." However, this fear is largely unfounded. Because of hormonal differences, it is very difficult for women to develop enormous muscles. Women bodybuilders require eight to ten years of intensive training to develop the prizewinning bodies we see on TV. Those muscles will never appear on an average woman who does a twenty-minute workout four times a week. But that twenty-minute strength-training session will have enormous benefits. Remember, increasing muscle tissue is the most reliable path to enhanced metabolism, greater energy, and effortless weight management.

Women who are interested in strength training can benefit from taking DHEA. DHEA actually helps replicate the energy level, confidence, and assertiveness of youth so that women, with proper training, can enjoy maximal workout techniques.

THE ULTIMATE MAXIMAL WORKOUT

The primary advantage of maximal training is time efficiency, and various companies have developed total-body aerobic machines designed to work both the upper and the lower body simultaneously. NordicTrack® is an excellent example, and there are numerous rowing machines that utilize leg resistance as well.

I thought my routine (twenty minutes of maximal training twice a week) was about as good as it gets until I was introduced to the ROM (short for range of motion) Time Machine. When I heard the manufacturer's claims of superior conditioning in four minutes a day, I was skeptical, to say the least. Conventional wisdom had placed the lower limit at about twenty minutes to achieve lasting cardiovascular benefits.

But the ROM machine delivered. In four minutes I had challenged to the max just about every muscle in my body. Afterward I felt as if I had performed forty-five minutes of maximal training: pleasantly exhausted but highly energized and mentally charged. I did what most people would do in that situation; I asked "How much?" The salesperson replied (with a straight face), "$10,400."

If that's a bit steep for you, you might try pleading with your health club to put one in the budget. They'll need plenty of space— the unit is an enormous (but beautiful) two-station Exercycle/ stair-climbing monster—but they'll also be impressed by a university study that backs up the manufacturer's claims.

Meanwhile, for those with no time, the four-minute total body workout is a reality . . . if you've got the bucks.

THE FORGOTTEN FACTORS: STRETCHING AND RELAXATION

No matter what your level of exercise, stretching may be the missing link to your success. Daily stretching will make all the difference in keeping your muscles and tendons limber as they adapt to your new routine.

Why don't more people stretch? Men don't stretch because they aren't good at it. Both men and women feel pressed for time and often opt for diving into the workout at hand, sometimes with painful results from tight muscles used too much, too soon. Set aside a mini-

STRENGTHEN AND STRETCH WITH YOGA

Yoga may be the most advanced system of stretching and toning ever developed. Yoga postures have the added advantage of increasing your flexibility and range of motion and strengthening your muscles and tendons by moving them in a variety of directions.

The nonforce movements of yoga are all natural and safe. This five-thousand-year-old practice can be undertaken by just about anyone. It is self-paced, and no special equipment is needed. While it is possible to learn yoga from books or videos, try to attend a class with a qualified yoga teacher, especially if you're just starting out. You'll experience benefits from the very first class, and those benefits will continue to build a strong and vibrant body for you.

mum of five to ten minutes a day for your stretching routine. This can consist of yoga postures or any other combination of stretches.

What about relaxation? Relaxation is definitely an important component of fitness. To get the maximum benefit from your program, be sure to take at least one day off per week. A day of rest will give your muscles the opportunity to rebuild themselves and become even stronger. As the intensity of your workouts increases to the maximal level, you will need to take off two days per week—one in midweek and one on the weekend—to continue reaping the greatest benefits.

YOUR FITNESS GOALS

What are your fitness goals? Do you want to feel better and have more energy? Are you trying to decrease body fat? Or are you ultimately interested in bodybuilding and maximal workouts?

Clearly defined fitness goals are the key to keeping up your motivation and building on your success. Take a few minutes to write out your specific fitness goals. Think in small increments and make your goals attainable. One example of a realistic, attainable goal is "I will walk for twenty minutes three days a week."

The goal "I want to lose twenty-five pounds" is too big to start with. If you have weight to lose, don't worry so much about the exact number of pounds. You'll drive yourself crazy and kill your motivation running to the bathroom scale every day. Just remember that there were no overweight cavemen or cavewomen. The DHEA Plan will put you back in sync with your genes and help you develop a youthful, powerful, energetic, and highly efficient body. As a result, your body weight will normalize, and even though weight loss may be slow (1 to 2 pounds a week is optimal), you'll be fitter than ever before and you'll keep the weight off.

Some people have a harder time reducing body fat because of genetics. If you want to lose weight, an important question to ask yourself is, "What is my genetic potential for that?" Set your goals accordingly. Strive to maximize your health, vitality, and fulfillment in life with whatever genes you have inherited along the way. I encourage people to reject the popular notion that equates beauty with an almost scarecrow thinness. Healthy bodies come in all sizes.

STAYING MOTIVATED

The key to keeping your motivation up is to design an exercise program that suits you. In addition to setting realistic goals, ask yourself the following questions:

- What am I willing to do to achieve my fitness goals?
- In order to exercise, do I need to make an appointment with a trainer?
- Would I prefer to exercise alone?
- Would I prefer to exercise with a friend or in a class?
- What rewards can I give myself for sticking with my program (new walking shoes, a new workout outfit, etc.)?

SEEK EXPERT ADVICE

If you are carrying extra weight or have a medical condition that requires special attention, see your physician before beginning an exercise program. If at all possible, hire a certified fitness trainer, especially if you are new to exercise. Enlist the help of a physical therapist for problems that require specially designed exercises.

Remember, the beauty of exercise is that people who are just starting out see the biggest results in the shortest period of time. You have nothing to lose and a world of vitality to gain by starting your exercise program today.

BIBLIOGRAPHY

Devlin JT, Horton ES. Metabolic fuel utilization during postexercise recovery. *Am J Clin Nutr* 1989; 49:944–8.

Goldfarb A, McIntosh M, Boyer B, Fatouros J. Vitamin E effects on indexes of lipid peroxidation in muscle from DHEA-treated and exercised rats. *J Appl Physiol* 1994; 76(4):1630–5.

Heath GW, Gavin JR, Hinderliter JM, Hagberg JM, Bloomfield SA, Holloszy JO. Effects of exercise and lack of exercise on glucose tolerance and insulin sensitivity. *J Appl Physiol* 1983; 55:512–7.

Jakubowicz D, Beer N, Rengifo R. Effect of dehydroepiandrosterone on cyclic-guanosine monophosphate in men of advancing age. *Ann NY Acad Sci* 1995; 774:312–5.

Yen SS, Morales AJ, Khorram O. Replacement of DHEA in aging men and women: Potential remedial effects. *Ann NY Acad Sci* 1995; 774:128–42.

CHAPTER 8

DHEA and Weight Management: How to Look Good in Your Genes

Your body type is controlled by genetics to a certain extent. If your ancestors were stocky, you'll tend to be stocky as well. Yet even within the confines of your genes there exists the potential for significant change. This is good news for the 60 percent of American adults who are overweight. You can feel better, look better, and achieve your optimum weight—starting today.

Overweight adults are the misunderstood majority. Every day more than 90 million Americans try to lose weight. Each year they spend over $30 billion on weight-loss products and programs. But despite their best efforts, few dieters are successful. Why?

If it were simply a matter of balancing calories in with calories out, weight loss would be a piece of cake. It's much more complex than that for most adults, because the actual balancing mechanism, the metabolism, is out of whack. As we grow older, our metabolism slows down and becomes less efficient. Many factors are involved, including stress, suboptimal nutrition, an overly processed diet, lack of exercise, and pollutants in the environment.

Enter DHEA. Restoring DHEA to prime peak levels is the next frontier for Americans seeking to lose weight. When combined with the proven strategies described in this chapter, DHEA can help transform your weight-loss program from fantasy to reality.

THE LEANNESS EFFECT

There is plenty of scientific evidence that DHEA helps reduce body fat. One study observed the effect of DHEA on genetically obese mice. The DHEA-treated mice ate normally but achieved and maintained thinness; they also lived longer than the control mice. In another study, when middle-aged obese rats were given DHEA-supplemented food, they lost weight.

This "leanness" effect has also been observed in studies involving humans. In fact, a study with human volunteers in 1988 showed that DHEA supplementation resulted in a 31 percent reduction in the percentage of body fat in 28 days. Isn't that what every dieter has always wanted and never experienced? Now it's possible.

Studies regarding DHEA and appetite show mixed results: Different experiments have shown increased, decreased, and unchanged appetite levels. Fat consumption seems to be a determining factor. DHEA-treated rats on a high-fat diet ate less than control rats did, while those on a low-fat diet ate more. But no matter what or how much they ate, the rats given DHEA consistently lost weight. The potential for weight loss in humans is truly exciting.

THE GLUCOSE CONNECTION

Obesity is inextricably tied to the insulin levels in your body. Insulin causes the body to store calories. When insulin levels are too high, it's just about impossible to lose weight. How do your insulin levels get that high in the first place? It happens when you try to control your glucose levels—no easy task, given the amounts of sugar most people ingest.

Sugar is almost pure glucose, and our bodies aren't designed to handle it. Remember that sugar is a very recent invention in the context of our evolution. For millennia the only sweets we had were complex starches that released glucose slowly into the bloodstream as they were digested. Today the average American eats more glucose in one day than our ancestors consumed in two weeks. And it's not just the amount but the speed at which this glucose enters the bloodstream.

Because sugar is such a refined simple carbohydrate, it is broken down by the enzymes in your saliva, so that chewing on a candy bar, for example, will start to raise your blood glucose (blood sugar) before you swallow the first bite. With today's refined and processed foods, blood sugar levels can rise very high and very fast.

What happens next? This spike in blood sugar causes the pancreas to kick in and secrete insulin to bring your glucose level back down. The problem is that the insulin response matches the intensity of the glucose load, often resulting in *excess* insulin secretion. A short time later you experience low blood sugar, otherwise known as hypoglycemia, Fog City, depression. Not only are you disoriented and craving sweets again, but the insulin response alerts your body to store that energy as fat.

THE ADRENAL RESPONSE

A healthy person gets out of Fog City with the aid of the adrenal glands. When blood sugar levels fall too far or too fast, the adrenals secrete stress hormones that cause the liver to release glucose into the bloodstream. That brings everything back to normal . . . in a healthy person.

However, we know from studies of DHEA that illness and aging can greatly affect adrenal function. As we grow older, this response may be slow, leaving us to languish in a hypoglycemic funk. Since that's quite uncomfortable, it's only natural that people take matters into their own hands. But what do we reach for? Either some more sugar or the adrenal kick in the pants known as caffeine. Either way, it simply starts the roller coaster ride all over again.

It's important to understand that this metabolic roller coaster shown in the chart on page 156 further weakens the adrenals, creating a vicious cycle of fluctuating blood sugar levels (with the associated mood and energy swings), hyperinsulin response, and stress. The irony is that while our bodies fight the "blood sugar wars," the majority of the calories ingested are being stored as fat. Why? Because weak adrenals cannot produce DHEA, and low DHEA means trouble.

DHEA actually inhibits one of the enzymes responsible for turning glucose into fat. This enzyme, G6PDH, determines to a great extent the fate of glucose molecules in your body. Research with animals has found that raising the DHEA level redirects glucose from fatstorage to energy-producing pathways, producing a leaner metabo-

THE INSULIN STRESS ROLLER COASTER

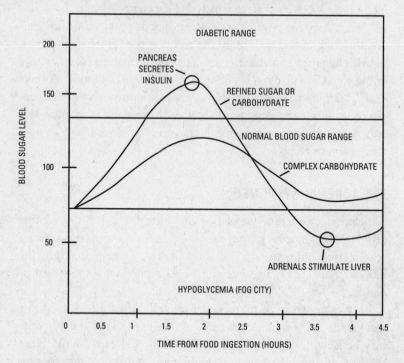

lism. DHEA is certainly not a "diet pill" and longer human studies still need to be done, but this exciting news may explain why men and women given supplemental DHEA for six months showed significant increases in muscle mass without making any changes in diet or exercise.

The second DHEA connection relates to insulin resistance, a common disorder that accompanies (and contributes to) obesity. As people age, especially if they also gain excess weight, the tissues become less sensitive to insulin. Since insulin is required to move glucose (fuel) out of the blood and into the cells, the body tries to compensate for this defect by producing more insulin. But since the underlying defect tends to worsen, all that is accomplished is that blood levels of insulin rise to dangerous heights. This condition, called *hyperinsulinemia* (medicalspeak for "too much insulin in the blood"), is a contributing factor in heart disease, hypertension, diabetes, and obesity.

Can you see the vicious cycle here? People fall into a sedentary lifestyle in their late twenties. They gain weight, and by the time they turn thirty, they are producing too much insulin. What's more, the excess fat on their bodies actually causes further insulin resistance, causing them to gain more weight. As they grow older, the condition only gets worse. These people can go on a hundred diets and fail every time because the metabolic deck is stacked against them. The only chance of success is to correct the underlying insulin defect, but that's a catch-22, because the only way to fix the insulin defect is to lose weight, and the only way to lose weight is to fix the insulin defect.

THE CATCH-23

DHEA can do much for an overweight person. As was mentioned above, its inhibition of G6PD may provide a significant metabolic adjustment from fat storage toward energy production. What's more, we know that increasing DHEA results in greater production of the muscle-building growth factor known as IGF-1. But as insulin levels rise, DHEA levels tend to fall. Dr. John Nestler and his colleagues at the Medical College of Virginia have shown that elevated insulin decreases DHEA production and increases the rate at which that substance is cleared from circulation. This would appear to seal the fate of anyone over age thirty trying to lose a significant amount of weight. However, there is light at the end of the tunnel, and once again it appears to be a torch carried by our Paleolithic ancestors.

WHY DIETS FAIL

Conventional diets fail because our bodies are finely tuned survival mechanisms. The job of our bodies is to stay alive, and we have developed incredible ways to adapt to even the harshest environments. One danger we have faced regularly in our history on earth is starvation, and so evolution designed a system to help us survive when food is scarce.

Similar to the hibernation response in bears, this "starvation response" causes our bodies to slow down and conserve calories whenever our caloric intake drops significantly. Thus, every time we start a new diet, our bodies say, "Uh oh, looks like a famine; time to slow down and store calories. Better make as much fat as possible . . . never know how long this will last."

The more we cut calories, the more our bodies try to slow down. Eventually, even though we're subsisting on a few lettuce leaves, our weight loss plateaus. We're so weak, hungry, and frustrated that we give up. Of course, when we start eating again, we end up gaining back even more weight than we lost.

CONVENTIONAL DIET BLUES

For over twenty years I have helped athletes, both professional and amateur, achieve high levels of performance. I've also assisted people who wanted to increase their level of fitness, lose weight, or just generally feel better. From 1975 to 1984 I counseled over nine thousand patients, using the prevailing wisdom of that time—what we now call "conventional" diets. I watched dedicated, hardworking people fail to achieve their goals in spite of their efforts, and I became increasingly depressed at the meager, short-lived success of my clients.

I talked to professional colleagues who were experiencing similar levels of frustration and failure and discovered that not even the bariatric specialists (physicians specializing in obesity and weight loss) were having much success. Challenged by the complexity of this problem and knowing that there had to be another way, I left clinical practice and went back into research.

DIET MYTHS DEBUNKED

I soon realized that the entire weight-loss industry had been constructed on false assumptions, and the biggest one was that weight loss is simply a matter of calories. I knew from my own experience that overweight people are neither lazy nor overindulgent. In reality, they are some of the most motivated and hardworking people around.

I found research that clearly refuted accusations of gluttony, including studies showing that many overweight individuals routinely consume fewer calories than do their thin counterparts. And the more

I dug into obesity research, the more I realized that dieters were laboring under not one but two burdens. In addition to excess weight, they were fighting against the mistaken assumptions on which every low-calorie diet was based. Here are some of those assumptions.

"METABOLISM ISN'T AN ISSUE." Wrong. While it is true that less than 3 percent of the population has "glandular" problems, I discovered other well-defined metabolic defects that had been completely overlooked.

"ALL CALORIES ARE THE SAME." Wrong. Low-calorie diets are still regarded as some sort of holy grail. The key is not the number of calories but what they consist of. Not only is there a definite difference in the way calories behave, but the body also goes into a "starvation response" on 1,200 calories or less a day unless it is "tricked" into a different response.

"ALL FAT IS BAD." Wrong. Some fats are absolutely essential for optimal health, and some types can actually stimulate the metabolic production of energy, creating more available energy and avoiding the storage of excess calories as body fat.

"REGULAR EXERCISE IS A MATTER OF WILLPOWER." Wrong. For many unfit people even minimal levels of exercise can leave them feeling exhausted, washed out, and depressed. Fortunately, there are natural ways to improve energy and stamina so that exercise is enjoyable and invigorating.

These false assumptions form the basis for conventional diets. However, since conventional diets have a 95 percent failure rate, it's time we realized that something's wrong with the diets, not the dieters. At the core of this failure is what I call the great diet myth: *the idea that simply reducing calories can result in permanent weight loss.* Nothing could be further from the truth.

In the past few years the idea that "diets don't work" has became commonplace. People have finally realized there must be something wrong, given the high failure rate. The weight-loss industry started talking about "programs" rather than "diets," but most are *still* based on the same false assumptions.

Through the DHEA Plan you can achieve your optimum weight with only a *moderate* reduction in calories. By combining prime peak levels of DHEA with bioenergetics and a connective tissue support program (see Chapter 6), along with regular exercise, you'll experience results that will surpass your greatest expectations.

BODY IMAGE: A MATTER OF PERCEPTION?

Dieting is often prompted by our perceptions of "ideal" weight. Consider the following:

- In a study of college women, 40 percent overestimated their body size.
- Twenty-five percent of men are constant dieters.
- Fifty percent of women are constant dieters.
- Ninety percent of teenage girls are unhappy with their weight, while only 13 percent actually exceed the standard weight for their height and body type.
- A point to ponder: What's your ideal weight? Who says?

For decades the height and weight tables of a life insurance company defined who was fit and who was fat. The table did not allow sufficiently for bone structure and lifestyle differences. The government recently issued new guidelines for "healthy weight" that are much more realistic. Here are the new guidelines:

GUIDELINES FOR HEALTHY WEIGHT
(without shoes or clothes)

Height	Age 19–34	35 and over
5'0"	97–128	108–138
5'1"	101–132	111–143
5'2"	104–137	115–148
5'3"	107–141	119–152
5'4"	111–146	122–157
5'5"	114–150	126–162
5'6"	118–155	130–167
5'7"	121–160	134–172
5'8"	125–164	138–178
5'9"	129–169	142–183
5'10"	132–174	146–188

5'11"	136–179	151–194
6'0"	140–184	155–199
6'1"	144–189	159–205
6'2"	148–195	164–210
6'3"	152–200	168–216
6'4"	156–205	173–222

METABOLIC FACTORS

For decades we've been told that except in rare cases, metabolism has nothing to do with being overweight. This absurd position holds that we all have high metabolic efficiency and that the only reason some people are thinner than others is because they eat less or exercise more. Pure rubbish!

You can look at your friends and family members and see that that's not true. Studies show that many overweight individuals consume fewer calories than do their normal-weight counterparts, often far fewer calories. Until they deal with the underlying metabolic factors, these people will never be able to achieve their ideal weight no matter how long they diet. As a matter of fact, the longer they diet, the farther they will be from their goal.

Many people want to lose weight, but few want to live in a deprived, malnourished state, consuming 800 to 1,000 calories a day. Our real goal is to feel better, look better, and enjoy life without being preoccupied with every bite we take. By improving our metabolic efficiency, we can reach our ideal weight while eating normal quantities of food and feeling healthy and energetic.

Through two decades of working with Olympic athletes, Hollywood celebrities, and weight-management programs, I've observed vast differences in eating programs, exercise habits, and weight levels. The differences I saw told me that there had to be metabolic factors that were being overlooked or ignored. That prompted me to conduct an exhaustive search through several thousand medical and scientific studies. This search revealed that obesity is a metabolic disorder and that control of metabolic factors is critical to the success of any long-term weight-management program.

The problem is that most "diets" involve deprivation ... and deprivation definitely does not work. You'll never have to count calories again if you take the appropriate steps to restore your metabolic efficiency to its optimum level.

NINE METABOLIC FACTORS IN WEIGHT LOSS

Most people in the modern world suffer from low metabolic efficiency, which leads to low fitness levels, sluggishness, fatigue, depression, apathy, excess fat, and a generally lowered appreciation of life. Obesity is a complex condition that often is aggravated by eating habits and self-esteem issues. The first step in reaching one's ideal weight is curing the metabolic imbalances caused by a sedentary lifestyle, poor food choices, and suboptimal nutrition.

Here are the nine metabolic factors in weight control:

1. APPETITE CONTROL SWITCH. When you eat a meal, a whole cascade of biochemical reactions takes place to digest, absorb, and metabolize the food. One of these reactions is the secretion of a hormone called *cholecystokinin* (CCK), which is produced by the small intestine. As CCK levels increase, your desire to eat decreases. Overweight individuals frequently have delayed secretion of CCK. When they eat, the appetite is switched off too late and overeating becomes an everyday experience.

The secretion of CCK takes place when partially digested proteins reach the small intestine, about fifteen to twenty minutes after the beginning of a meal. A fast eater can consume an incredible number of calories before enough CCK is secreted to turn off the appetite. The obvious answer is to eat more slowly. Or try this: Eat a whole raw carrot or a cup of hot soup at the beginning of a meal. This naturally slows you down, allowing time for the secretion of CCK. You feel more satisfied with fewer calories.

2. ESSENTIAL FATS. Not all fats are bad. Most Americans consume too much fat, but the *type* of fat you eat is as important as the amount. Some fats are absolutely essential for human health, and some fats can help you lose weight. Essential fats come from vegetable sources (beans, nuts, seeds, olives) and cold-water fish such as salmon, mackerel, and Icelandic cod. Nonessential fats come from animal sources (meat, chicken, eggs, dairy products).

If you have ever experienced changes in your skin and hair when dieting (dry, scaly skin and brittle or dull hair), chances are that you were malnourished in essential fats. Essential fat deficiency produces metabolic problems that actually inhibit weight loss. If you don't eat sufficient amounts of essential fats, you can actually gain weight.

3. OXYGEN. The only way to get rid of fat is by burning it to create energy. Our energy fires require lots of oxygen. To keep those fires burning, we need an efficient oxygen delivery system. This requires a high level of aerobic fitness—a strong heart, lungs, and muscles—exactly what most overweight people don't have.

In spite of the "no pain, no gain" mentality, studies show that exercising to the point of exhaustion is disastrous to weight-loss goals. When we reach exhaustion, the body's oxygen stores are depleted and it is forced to burn primarily protein (muscle), glucose (blood sugar), and a stored form of glucose called glycogen. This produces hypoglycemia (low blood sugar), resulting in fatigue, depression, and a ravenous desire for sweets. So by all means exercise, but be moderate enough to avoid the huffing and puffing signs of oxygen debt.

Gradually you'll be able to increase the intensity and duration of your exercise program. Chapter 7 explains exactly how to do so sensibly and with ease.

4. THE FAT "ESCORT." The fat in your body doesn't volunteer to be burned. Fat-burning enzymes must be produced to "escort" the fat molecules to the energy factories in your muscles. Exercise stimulates the production of these fat-burning enzymes, but the critical factor in this case is *duration*. Research shows that increased enzyme production begins after about thirty minutes of moderate exercise, but most overweight people run out of steam before they reach that threshold. This makes exercise a continuous struggle and keeps fat-burning at a minimum. No wonder we get discouraged.

The DHEA Plan helps you increase your exercise tolerance by correcting nutrient deficiencies and gives you a specific exercise program to stimulate the production of fat-burning enzymes (see Chapter 7).

5. INSULIN RESISTANCE. For the past thirty years medical experts have been aware of the relationship between obesity and insulin. Insulin is a hormone involved in the delivery of fuel to the cells of the body. Most overweight people suffer from some degree of insulin resistance, which impairs the delivery of fuel. This results in fatigue, low exercise tolerance, and decreased fat-burning. As was explained earlier in this chapter, DHEA, diet, and regular exercise can all help stabilize insulin levels to make weight loss easier.

6. THE STARVATION RESPONSE. When one lowers one's calorie intake dramatically, the body thinks it has entered a time of famine. Some studies show that low-calorie diets can reduce the metabolic rate by as much as 36 percent. The body slows down, conserves fat stores, and waits for the famine to end. And when it does, it's feast time. We pile our plates high, and our bodies gear up for massive fat storage. We call this the *yo-yo diet syndrome*, and the normal result is that we lose weight and then gain back even more. It seems like a cruel joke, but it's really just our bodies being superefficient.

7. THE ENEMY ENZYME. There is one enzyme no one in the weight-loss industry seems to be talking about—lipoprotein lipase (LPL). Regardless of how long you've struggled or how much weight you've lost, LPL can make you fat again. It's not fair, but it's the truth. It's another survival mechanism. LPL grabs fat molecules and warehouses them on your thighs, around your middle, and in other jiggly storage areas in your body.

Without knowing how to regulate LPL, the deck is heavily stacked against you and long-term weight management is difficult. Conventional diets elevate LPL levels, and those levels can stay elevated up to six months after the diet has ended. No wonder weight comes back so fast.

It is critical that your body not think it's being starved or deprived. Certain foods naturally help lower the level of LPL in fat tissue. These foods help you feel full and satisfied and keep your body from approaching the starvation response. We'll talk more about these foods later in this chapter.

8. TIMING. A Chinese proverb states: "In all things watch the timing." This is as true in weight management as it is in all other life endeavors. Research shows that the timing of food intake has much to do with what happens to the ingested calories. Going without adequate calories even for only four or five hours can trigger the starvation response and raise LPL. That means that calories consumed after the "famine" will be stored as fat as the body prepares to face another round of starvation. Skipping breakfast or lunch and rewarding ourselves with a high-calorie dinner is a recipe for failure and frustration.

YOUR ENERGY WAREHOUSE MANAGER

Deep within your brain is an energy warehouse manager that is in charge of cataloging and shipping fuel throughout your body. This energy manager has been working in your body for quite some time and has developed a thorough understanding of your energy needs. The manager knows about how much energy you will need during the day, and that amount is stored primarily as glycogen, which is easily converted to energy. Any excess calories that come in are stored as fat.

Unfortunately for us, the energy manager has an expandable warehouse for fat but not for glycogen, which can only be stored in the liver and muscles. The DHEA Plan helps you maximize glycogen production and storage, empowering you with greater energy and reducing the storage of fat.

The timing of food intake, activity, and exercise is extremely important. Your brain takes cues from your muscles about what to do with calories: store them as glycogen (a form of energy) or as fat. Every time you add activity to your routine, you're sending a signal that this is an active body and more glycogen (and less fat) should be kept on hand. Long hours in front of the television send a message that the body doesn't need energy, and calories are converted to fat. The DHEA Plan shows you how to increase your exercise and activity levels in ways that will send your metabolism fat-avoiding messages.

9. MIND AND METABOLISM. Numerous studies of athletes have proved that mental imagery stimulates physical responses in the body. If mentally picturing a specific result can increase muscle strength and improve athletic performance, I thought, why not use it to stimulate metabolic efficiency and aid weight loss? Mental imagery can be a powerful tool in a weight-loss program. Your mind can be a powerful ally in stimulating CCK, decreasing the enemy enzyme LPL, and maintaining your motivation and attitude toward fitness. We'll talk more about mental imagery at the end of this chapter.

FROM INFORMATION TO ACTION

Understanding obesity in its evolutionary context—it is a survival response encoded in our Paleolithic genes—enables us to focus on the root cause (metabolism) and not simply the symptom (too many pounds). Is there a way to reduce caloric intake without triggering this survival response of lowered metabolic rate and increased fat storage? Finally, the answer is yes, but you'll need a number of important tools.

THE DIETER'S ESSENTIAL BAG OF TRICKS

- **FIBER**—enhances stomach fullness, delays stomach emptying.
- **ADEQUATE PROTEIN**—stimulates production of CCK, the body's appetite "off" switch; helps balance excess carbohydrate to avoid raising insulin levels.
- **MEDIUM-CHAIN TRIGLYCERIDES (MCTS)**—prevent stimulation of LPL and provide energy.
- **GARCINIA EXTRACT**—helps control appetite and decreases the conversion of calories to fat.
- **DESERT CACTUS**—contains starches that provide energy without stimulating insulin.
- **BIOENERGETICS**—are vital, and it would be a good idea to go back to Chapter 7 and review the section on bioenergetics. These essential nutrients, including coenzyme Q10, chromium, and alpha-ketoglutaric acid, can dramatically improve your body's production of energy on every level. This not only makes exercise easier and more enjoyable but *enhances the benefits that you receive from exercise.* What's more, scientists have found that correcting a chromium insufficiency can dramatically improve insulin metabolism. For the dieter, optimal bioenergetic nutrition is an absolute must.

The next section will help you understand each of these tools and how they provide the metabolic advantage that will allow you to lose weight easily and naturally.

FABULOUS FIBER

Fiber is a wonderful diet food. Since it is indigestible, it contains no calories. Fiber expands, giving you a sense of fullness, and helps regulate blood sugar. The benefits of fiber have been discussed widely in the past few years, yet studies show that most Americans consume far less than the recommended level of dietary fiber. The bad news is that it's almost impossible to reach the recommended levels of fiber in today's processed foods.

Most of the recent fiber news has focused on wheat bran and oat bran. These are both excellent sources of fiber, but so are rice bran and gum fibers. Fiber slows the rate at which food leaves the stomach, thus maintaining the fullness effect. What's more, gum fiber such as guar and other sources such as psyllium contain mostly *soluble* fiber, which has been proven effective in reducing blood cholesterol levels.

One simple way to increase the fiber in your diet is to take a shaker container with large holes (similar to a Parmesan cheese container) and fill it with a cup of wheat bran mixed with a half cup of oat bran and a quarter cup of rice bran (all available in health food stores). Shake this mixture on everything: breakfast cereal, salads, mashed potatoes, and especially soup. Each tablespoon will give you approximately 3 grams of dietary fiber (equally divided between soluble and insoluble), and it should not be difficult to consume two tablespoons through the course of your day.

POWERFUL PROTEIN

The *amount* of protein that is best for weight loss is a matter of debate. I'll give you my Paleolithic perspective later in this chapter, but right now I want to talk about the fact that protein stimulates the secretion of CCK better than fats or carbohydrates. A trick I've used quite successfully with clients (especially those who eat fast) is to consume a small amount of predigested protein right before meals. There are literally dozens of protein supplement options available today, including powders, liquids, tablets, and chewable wafers. What you're looking for is a semi-digested or predigested product that will give you 8 to 10 grams of protein. Don't spend a lot of money on free-form amino acids. Products containing large protein fragments known as peptides work even better and cost less. Even in such small quantities these proteins are powerful CCK stimulators. They also stimulate another hormone, called *gastrin*, which may improve digestion.

MEDIUM-CHAIN TRIGLYCERIDES

Through the years the overweight people I have counseled have been on many diets; some have tried twenty or more. Although they weren't aware of it, each diet triggered an elevation of LPL, which created a *fat-forming* metabolism that made successful weight management virtually impossible. To a great extent, LPL is responsible for every bulge on your body, but this monster can be tamed.

While you would think that someone would have figured this out before now, maybe it was too obvious. LPL is a survival mechanism that helps the body deal with starvation. It is triggered by the drastic reduction in calories that is typical of all conventional diets. Therefore, the assumption was that nothing could be done about LPL. However, when you look carefully at the research, you find that there is a natural substance that prevents the elevation of LPL—and that substance is fat.

Fat calories send a message that the body is *not* starving, so LPL is not increased. However, in a weight-loss program the type of fat is critical. We need a fat that will keep the LPL monster happy without winding up on our thighs. Amazingly enough, there *is* such a fat, and it's known as MCTs. Relatively small amounts of MCTs will tell your body that it's not being deprived, and this will cancel one important component of the starvation response.

But MCTs are even more special. Ordinary fats go through a multistage digestion process, after which they travel to the liver, where they are utilized or stored as fat, according to the body's efficiency. Since overweight people have low metabolic efficiency, a large percentage winds up in the fat storehouses.

MCTs, however, are digested in one easy step and are absorbed directly into the bloodstream. These energy-rich particles go to the liver or are absorbed directly by the working muscles or other tissues, where they are easily burned to fulfill the body's energy needs. MCTs are not stored as fat except by the most sedentary body. Thus, MCTs deliver highly efficient energy and prevent the starvation response by taming the LPL monster.

You can find MCTs in the bodybuilding or sports area of a health food store. MCTs are used by endurance athletes to help fuel strenuous workouts and marathon-length competition. Look for pure MCTs rather than a megaproduct containing every nutrient known. Pure MCTs are available in oil and capsule form, and you only need 3 or 4 grams (one tablespoon) a day to be effective. MCT oil, which has a neutral taste, can be added to salad dressing and soup, poured on toast, or taken like medicine.

Garcinia Extract

The herb *Garcinia cambogia* has been used for centuries as an aid to weight loss. It can help reduce hunger and has been shown to decrease the synthesis of fat by the liver. The active ingredient in the herb is a compound known as hydroxycitric acid (HCA), so it is important to purchase a product that contains a known quantity of this ingredient. Most major brands utilize standardized extracts providing 50 percent HCA. Garcinia is available today in a wide variety of tablets, liquids, and powders. A garcinia chewing gum may be available soon. Remember that these products are most effective when taken between meals and that the benefits are cumulative. Thus, it is better to take garcinia three or four times a day rather than all at once. The dose that appears to be effective is somewhere between 1500 and 3000 mg of garcinia per day, yielding 750 to 1500 mg of HCA. Less than 1500 mg may not provide the hunger satisfaction you desire.

It's important to note that garcinia is not an appetite suppressant. Drugs that have commonly been used to suppress appetite do so by making you slightly sick to your stomach. The result is that you don't (or can't) eat, which is great for short-term weight loss but disastrous for long-term success. That's because drastic calorie reduction triggers drastic starvation responses in your body. The secret is to reduce calories *moderately* while you tune up your metabolism and begin regular and consistent exercise. Garcinia can be an invaluable aid because it doesn't make food impossible to eat. You still enjoy your meals; it's just that you find that you are satisfied with eating less. Together with the protein-CCK "trick," most people find that it's easy to decrease calories 20 to 30 percent and report feeling satisfied, comfortable, and energized at the same time. Isn't that the kind of "diet" you want?

THE CACTUS CONNECTION

The last trick you may need is one that I came upon by accident. I was scanning through research concerning glucose metabolism and came across data from Mexico and South America identifying a certain cactus (botanical name: *Opuntia streptacantha*; common name: prickly pear) that has been used traditionally as a treatment for diabetes. Curious about how a cactus could modify blood sugar, I pored through a number of botanical texts and learned that this cactus contains a simple, easily digested starch that does not stimulate insulin secretion.

Here's how that fits into the weight-loss puzzle. I've described the fat component of the starvation response and how it can be canceled by taking MCTs. However, there's also a blood sugar component, which means that when the brain runs low on glucose, it presses the emergency button. Researchers had long sought a starch that would send glucose to the brain without triggering the insulin roller coaster described earlier, and here it is.

Since this discovery a few manufactures have incorporated cactus concentrate into their weight-loss products. The benefit? It allows you to decrease calories but maintain a positive mood and a clear head. Most important, the message from the brain to the body is this: "Hey, there's fewer calories coming in today, but everything up here is cool. If you guys (muscles and other tissues) need more energy . . . burn some fat."

A THIN STYLE OF EATING

In Japan a man who weighed well over four hundred pounds asked my advice on how to *gain* weight! He was a sumo wrestler, and I was there doing research on bioenergetics. My host, a Japanese scientist, had invited me to see the sumo contest and meet some of the wrestlers, who are enormous men, often weighing over five hundred pounds. I was astonished to learn that their diet was pretty much the same as the normal low-fat Japanese diet: rice, vegetables, soybeans, and fish.

How did these men gain so much weight on a diet we use to help people lose weight? When I asked my host that question, he replied with a smile, "Timing."

In spite of my host's cryptic comment, I was surprised when later conversations with the wrestlers showed a pattern of weight gain that depended not so much on *what* they ate as on *when* they ate and what they did afterward. One wrestler explained the typical sumo training schedule:

Morning	Workout
Noon	Lunch meal
Afternoon	Nap (three hours or more)
Evening	Main meal
Night	Snacks

Sumo Wrestlers Skip Breakfast

When I asked about breakfast, the wrestler said, "We never eat breakfast. Only lunch and dinner and snacks later on." Of course, these wrestlers were consuming large quantities of food, but I was intrigued by the question of timing. Did it really matter that much *when* they ate?

As soon as I returned to my office in Los Angeles, I began to look into research on meal frequency and metabolism. As it turned out, scientists were just beginning to understand what sumo wrestlers had known for centuries: Timing is a major factor in building fat. The primary difference is between two styles of eating—nibbling and gorging.

Sumo wrestlers gorge. They skip breakfast, which means they go for about fifteen hours without eating, and then they consume large quantities of food at two sittings. The long period without food primes the body's starvation response and raises the level of LPL. Then, when the first big meal is consumed, the body goes into a fat storage mode.

Another factor in the sumo wrestlers' massive size is the way they work out. In the ring they're involved in explosive movement, but otherwise they sit on the sidelines and watch. This on and off activity burns glycogen, not fat. The sumo workout actually intensifies the "store fat" messages going to their bodies.

After a large lunch, which their bodies see as the feast that follows a famine, sumo wrestlers take a long nap. And then, after that long period of inactivity, comes another big meal. This activity pattern sends a strong message to the warehouse manager in the brain: "This body is inactive; the muscles don't need energy, so store as much as possible as fat."

RESEARCH YIELDS HEFTY RESULTS

Thirty years ago a group of researchers noted that individuals consuming a few large meals tended to be overweight, whereas lean subjects ate approximately the same number of calories in smaller, more frequent feedings. This was an intriguing association, but was there a cause-and-effect relationship between meal frequency and obesity? That answer came in the 1970s when researchers identified specific metabolic changes that occur as a result of gorging behavior. The most important effect was increased deposition of fat, referred to as *adaptive hyperlipogenesis* (*hyper*, "excessive"; *lipo*, "fat"; *genesis*, "formation"). Research in rats showed that gorging resulted in weight gain, even when they ate 25 percent fewer calories than the nibbling group.

FOLLOWING THE SUMO DIET

As fascinating as it was to understand how sumo wrestlers achieve their enormous size, it was even more astounding to realize that most of us follow the same pattern in America, especially if we're dieting and trying to lose weight.

Think about it. Many dieters skip breakfast or consume a very light breakfast (200 calories or less). Morning activity often consists of sitting at a desk with maybe a bit of walking, carrying a briefcase, or lifting a laundry basket. Lunch is the first "real" meal of the day, and it is followed by three or four more hours of inactivity (sitting at a desk or in a classroom, watching television, etc.). And then, after all this inactivity, we consume a large evening meal, followed by more inactivity and often some snacks. *You couldn't design a better way to gain weight if you tried.*

FROM GORGING TO GRAZING

So what to do? If we want to lose weight, we need to switch from gorging to grazing. Research shows that consuming smaller, more frequent meals sends an entirely different message to the brain: "There is a reliable inflow of calories; there's no risk of starvation; calories can be stored as glycogen rather than fat."

If you add consistent, moderate-intensity exercise to this behavior, the message becomes even better: "This is an active body; better break down some stored fat and send energy to the muscles." And, if you add some upper body strength training to build muscle mass, the message to your brain is "This is an active, strong, and dynamic body with a reliable inflow of calories. Maximize metabolic efficiency and get rid of all that unnecessary baggage (fat, toxins). Increase muscle metabolism and just burn up all that excess fat. Send as much energy as possible to every muscle, tissue, and organ."

This produces what is known as *vitality*: the natural fulfillment of the body's innate ability to experience peak performance on every level. Here are some of the benefits of reaching this level of vitality:

- A powerful and vigilant immune system
- A highly efficient respiratory and cardiovascular system delivering ample fat-burning oxygen to every cell and effectively removing metabolic debris
- A finely tuned nervous system managing stress easily and creating mental clarity
- Powerful muscles, tendons, ligaments, and joints, enabling you to move with invigorating confidence
- An efficient endocrine system producing an abundance of fat-burning enzymes, digestive enzymes, thyroid and growth hormones; improved glucose tolerance with a decreased risk for diabetes and hypoglycemia

MANAGING YOUR FATS

Americans typically obtain nearly 40 percent of their total calories from fat. This makes weight management extremely difficult, because the fat you eat can easily be added to the fat stored in your body. While carbohydrates and even protein can be converted to fat, that requires an energy-burning multistep process. In other words, your body burns calories to convert carbohydrates and protein to fat. Consumed fat, however, becomes part of your body's fat stores in the blink of an eye.

Decreasing fat in your diet starts with reducing highly saturated fats such as those found in meat, eggs, butter, cheese and other dairy products, mayonnaise, and salad dressings. However, to get your total fat down to the recommended level of 30 percent or less of total calories, you need to become a good "fat finder."

Read food labels to see how many grams of fat are in each serving. Beware of serving sizes; often they're much smaller than the serving size normally consumed. Multiply the number of fat grams by nine (the number of calories in each gram of fat) and you have the fat calories per serving. If it's over 60 calories, chances are that you're looking at a high-fat food.

You can divide the total fat calories by the total calories per serving to get the percentage of calories derived from fat. This is extremely valuable information because it gives you a clear and accurate idea of the food's weight-management value. Your goal is to keep this figure under 30 percent. While some foods consumed during the day may be higher than this number, your daily total should stay under 30 percent. The FDA has recommended that food manufacturers add this figure to their labels, and some do.

If the percentage of calories derived from fat is not on the label, be suspicious, and don't be deceived by the labels proclaiming "80 percent fat-free" or even "90 percent fat-free." This does not mean that these foods necessarily fall into your guidelines. Generally, these labels refer to percentage of fat *by weight*, not by calories. Here's how this works.

A national brand of turkey franks is advertised as being "80 percent fat-free." A quick look at the label reveals that each frank contains 11 grams of fat, or a total of 99 calories derived from fat. The total calories in each frank is only 130, which means that the actual percentage of fat is 76 percent. Would you say that's a misleading label? I think so, and your only defense is to become an educated label reader.

HIDDEN FAT

Here is a list of foods that will almost always exceed your 30 percent guidelines:

- Commercial baked goods, including crackers
- Cream soups, sauces, creams and gravies
- Candy, especially chocolates
- Nondairy coffee lightener
- Salad dressings and mayonnaise
- Peanuts and other nuts
- All fried foods
- Potato chips
- Popcorn (microwave or movie theater)
- Stuffing and packaged potato items
- Puddings and other desserts
- Breaded fish
- Quiche
- Pizza

JUST SAY NO TO SUGAR

All calories are not created equal, and sugar calories are some of the worst. Sugar not only contributes nutritionally worthless calories but also raises blood insulin levels. Since insulin is an anabolic (tissue-building) hormone, an increase in the insulin level sends a powerful message to every cell in the body to *store* calories. As I have already mentioned, excess insulin production is also responsible for lowering DHEA levels.

Sugar triggers your hunger mechanism. Here's how it works: Appetite is regulated in part by the level of glucose in the blood. When you eat a meal, the complex carbohydrates (vegetables, grains, beans, fruits) are broken down into glucose and absorbed into the blood-stream. This glucose is used to fuel all the life functions of the body, including growth, repair, brain function, and movement. Later, when blood glucose levels decline to the low-normal range, your hunger mechanism is stimulated. This is a normal four- to five-hour cycle.

Refined sugars throw this cycle off completely. Unlike complex carbohydrates, which require time to be digested, simple sugars release glucose into the bloodstream very quickly. In fact, when you eat a high-sugar food, glucose levels in the blood may rise in as little as fifty seconds. The body responds to the onslaught of sugar as a metabolic emergency and begins to secrete insulin, driving glucose out of the blood and into the cells. As a result, blood glucose levels can fall rapidly, creating another metabolic emergency.

You probably know what comes next. Not only do you feel tired and confused as your muscles and brain search for glucose, your hunger mechanism is stimulated even if you ate just twenty minutes before. This can lead to food cravings, binge eating, and a constant feeling of being out of control.

A good weight-loss program therefore will limit refined sugars and place more emphasis on protein and natural carbohydrates such as whole grains, beans, and vegetables. Fruits are fine if eaten as whole fruit. The difference, however, between an apple and a glass of apple juice is remarkable. The apple provides chewing satisfaction, fiber, and significant hunger satisfaction. It's a sensible snack. Apple juice contains concentrated fruit sugar and no fiber. It can easily throw you into the sugar-insulin roller coaster you're trying to avoid.

Adequate protein can also help put the brakes on the insulin roller coaster. High-carbohydrate meals such as pasta (usually served with bread) can raise insulin levels almost as much as sugar does. Try adding some protein at the beginning of the meal in the form of a low-fat or nonfat dairy product such as cottage cheese or use a protein supplement.

Note: Alcohol is metabolized by the body very much as sugar is. It not only raises insulin levels but also inhibits fat-burning enzymes. Make alcoholic beverages an occasional treat, not a regular part of your diet.

SUMO EATING VERSUS THIN EATING

Here's a quick test to see if your style of eating resembles that of a sumo wrestler:

— 1. Do you eat most of your calories in one or two large meals?
— 2. Is your largest meal in the evening?
— 3. Does your food intake vary greatly (weekend binging followed by several days of restrained eating)?

— 4. Do you frequently "diet" (follow a low-calorie eating plan) for a week or more at a time?

— 5. Are you sedentary after you eat (sitting at your desk or in front of the TV)?

— 6. Do you tend to eat more processed foods (snacks, white bread, refined cereals) than you do whole grains (brown rice, whole wheat bread, whole grain cereals)?

— 7. Do you eat more high-fat and high-sugar foods than you do fresh fruits and vegetables?

— 8. Do you eat fewer than five servings of fresh fruits and vegetables each day?

— 9. Do you eat fewer than five servings of whole grains, beans, and cereals each day?

— 10. Are you a fast eater?

— 11. Do you use caffeine or herbal stimulants to decrease your appetite and get you through the day?

A majority of "yes" answers to these questions indicates that you may eat more like a sumo wrestler than like a thin person. These habits unnecessarily maximize the conversion of calories to fat. The human body processes food differently depending on when you eat, how frequently you eat, how much is eaten at one time, how much fiber the meal contains, and what your activity level is during the day. Here are some important tips to developing a "thin" style of eating.

1. EAT SEVERAL SMALL MEALS. Studies show that eating four to five small meals will optimize digestion, improve metabolism, and reduce the conversion of calories to fat. Grazing is better than gorging.

2. AVOID SKIPPING MEALS. Going even four or five hours without food can trigger the starvation response and cause your metabolism to slow down.

3. REDUCE THE EVENING MEAL. When you eat, your metabolism increases to digest the food. Much of this increased energy is given off as heat. This thermogenic effect significantly reduces the amount of calories absorbed from a meal. It is much higher in the morning than it is at night. Studies show that when individuals consumed a large meal (650 calories) in the morning, they did not gain weight. When the same group consumed the large meal at night, 76 percent of them showed a significant weight gain.

4. EAT BEFORE EXERCISE. When you exercise on an empty stomach, the body, perceiving not only hunger but also activity, may further lower the metabolic rate. Eat a small meal or snack forty minutes to an hour before exercising.

5. REDUCE CALORIES GRADUALLY. If you go on a low-calorie diet, your body eliminates all or part of the thermogenic effect in an effort to conserve energy. In addition, enzymes are produced that signal the body to store all available calories as fat. These two survival mechanisms will not only sabotage weight loss but contribute to increased weight gain as soon as a normal diet is resumed.

6. EAT HIGH-FIBER FOODS. Consuming high-fiber foods such as whole grains, beans, vegetables, and fruits results in decreased fat storage. Not only are these foods naturally low in fat, but a portion of the fat consumed during a high-fiber meal is combined with the fiber and eliminated as waste.

7. AVOID HIGH-FAT FOODS. All calories are not created equal. Excess calories from fat will make you fat a great deal faster than will excess calories from protein or carbohydrates. The conversion of carbohydrates and protein to fat requires a great deal of energy. Fat calories, however, are easily converted to stored fat in your body.

8. DECREASE THE USE OF SUGARS. This means not only table sugar but also glucose, dextrose, brown sugar, corn syrup, high-fructose corn syrup, honey, molasses, and maple syrup. Sugar is a major enemy of weight control, adding worthless calories and sending a message to every cell in the body to store calories.

9. WHEN IN DOUBT, EAT VEGETABLES. Vegetables are the dieter's best friend, and I don't mean just carrot and celery sticks. Expand your vegetable intake to include a wide variety of delicious, high-energy foods from the produce section of the grocery store. Most markets offer some forty types of vegetables that can be steamed, broiled, barbecued, or eaten raw in a salad. Vegetables are low in calories and high in vitamins, minerals, and complex carbohydrates. Because they are an excellent source of fiber, vegetables also contribute to a sense of fullness and satisfaction.

10. SEND ACTIVITY MESSAGES. Studies show that your brain gets metabolic "signals" depending on your activity level during the day. Don't let your body forget that it is active and needs a high level of energy. Remember that calories do not evaporate. They must be stored as energy (glycogen) or as fat. For successful long-term weight management you must convince your body that you are active and need energy. Take frequent activity breaks every couple of hours. Ten minutes of brisk walking, a few flights of stairs, or a quick set of stretching exercises will do the trick. A longer activity break of fifteen to twenty minutes after meals is highly recommended. A moderate-paced thirty- to forty-minute walk will help to convert calories to energy rather than fat.

11. EAT SLOWLY. Appetite is regulated in part by the secretion of CCK. This hormone is released toward the end of a meal and sends a signal to the brain to shut off the appetite. Eating fast tends to bypass this important message, leading to the overconsumption of food. Adding protein to the beginning of a meal will help stimulate CCK and provide a natural feeling of satisfaction with surprisingly few calories.

12. AVOID STIMULANTS. Caffeine and herbal stimulants produce a stress response that temporarily suppresses your appetite. A few hours later, not only will your appetite be back with a vengeance, but your nervous system will be the worse for wear. There are no long-term studies indicating any weight-loss benefits from stimulants.

13. TAKE OUT SOME NUTRITION INSURANCE. Research shows that if a diet was *perfectly* planned, it would still take about 2,000 calories for men and 1,500 calories for women to provide them with a barely adequate level of vitamins and minerals. Since most of us don't have the time or energy to plan our meals perfectly, multivitamins are an effective form of "nutritional insurance." Since most dieters consume fewer calories than those perfect levels, it's easy to see why dieters have been called the nation's largest group of malnourished people.

The DHEA Plan encourages sensible eating and focuses on metabolic efficiency and exercise as the primary weight-loss tools. This approach not only avoids the starvation response that results in a lowering of the metabolic rate but also provides greater nutrient availability. However, I still highly recommend a quality multivitamin to fill in the gaps created by today's processed foods and fast-paced, stress-filled lifestyle.

14. DRINK WATER. Water can be a wonderful help in a weight-loss program. The water you drink is essential for the transport and burning of fat as well as the elimination of waste products that result from enhanced metabolic activity. In fact, water is vital to all the body's functions, including movement, digestion, and temperature regulation. Most people don't drink enough water and, as you begin to exercise more, you'll find that your need for water increases.

Don't rely on thirst. As it turns out, thirst is not a reliable indication of the need for water. Research shows that the body can become significantly dehydrated before we actually feel thirsty. To prevent this, we suggest that you develop a "water habit" that ensures the intake of eight to ten glasses per day.

If you're in one place most of the day, this will be easy. Simply take a 24-ounce tumbler and fill it up in the morning and be sure that it's empty by midmorning. Refill it and make sure that that's gone by midafternoon. The last 24 ounces should be consumed before 5 p.m. You will probably need to consume more water after your walk or workout.

The need for water does not always result in a clear signal to the brain. Sometimes we simply experience a vague physiological need and may interpret that signal as a call for food. Since most foods contain significant amounts of water, this practice generally fills our need for water, but we end up consuming too many calories. When we feel those vague cravings, our first response should be to drink a glass of water. If it was merely thirst, the water will satisfy the need.

Drinking enough water will reduce fluid retention and edema. It's sometimes hard for people to understand that drinking lots of water actually decreases water retention. However, if you provide your body with ample amounts of pure water, it will not have to retain water in the tissues. Other fluids, such as tea, juice, sodas, milk, and coffee, contain water, but they also contain many other ingredients, including diuretics (which cause you to lose water) and salt.

Diuretic drugs offer only a temporary solution to water retention. Your body will compensate for diuretics as soon as you stop taking them. The real solution to a water retention problem is to drink plenty of pure water. This makes it easy for your body to supply its metabolic needs and helps in the rapid elimination of waste. Adequate water also reduces the common experience of muscle aches and helps relieve constipation.

TIPS ON GETTING ENOUGH WATER

1. Always have a bottle of water handy and sip it all day.

2. Put a sign on the refrigerator that reads "Choose Water!"

3. Drink a glass of water slowly as you prepare your meal.

4. Remind yourself that the more water you drink, the better you will feel.

5. Do not keep soft drinks in your home.

6. Flavor your water with a squeeze of lemon or lime or with a small amount of fruit juice.

15. FORGET DIET FOODS, AND ESPECIALLY DIET SOFT DRINKS. According to a recent FDA report, Americans spent over $30 *billion* on diet foods and beverages in 1994, and sales are expected to grow to at least $35 billion by 1998. But while the diet food industry expands, so do the waistlines of 100 million Americans. That's because diet foods are not the solution. Advertisers would love you to believe that the svelte model sipping that diet cola was once overweight and became thin by drinking their beverage, but that is far from the truth. Advertisers would like you to believe that weight management is simply a matter of reducing calories, but you know better.

The belief that food *quality* doesn't matter as long as a food is low in calories is a dangerous misconception. Look carefully at diet food labels. You'll often find excessive salt, sweeteners, artificial colors and flavors, and ingredients you can't pronounce. Some of these ingredients are health risks, but we buy the products anyway because we are desperate to lose weight.

If the products worked, it might be worth the risk of ingesting all those chemicals, fake fats, artificial sweeteners, and stabilizers. *But the products don't work.* Bob Schwartz, the author of *Diets Don't Work*, was one of the first health experts to point out that the use of diet foods does not help individuals understand the cause of obesity any more than an aspirin helps someone understand the cause of a headache. In both cases the condition reappears until the root cause is dealt with.

The root cause of obesity, as I have explained, has to do with metabolism, energy, exercise, muscle mass, attitude, and food quality. Calories do count, but not much.

In fact, scientific studies show that the consumption of diet beverages may actually promote weight gain. In a six-year study of 80,000 women, researchers found that the habitual users of artificial sweeteners put on excess pounds. Artificial sweetener users were far more likely to gain weight than were women who didn't use them. Among all the women who gained weight, the users of artificial sweeteners gained significantly more weight than did the nonusers.

Why? Some researchers believe that while people may try to decrease their caloric intake by using diet foods, many make up for the decreased calories by eating twice as much or eating additional foods that they wouldn't normally consume. Biochemically, it may be that artificial sweeteners actually increase the appetite. In a blind study (the subjects did not know if they were consuming aspartame or sugar) the subjects receiving aspartame reported increased motivation to eat and decreased ratings of fullness.

Research also suggests that artificial sweeteners can create a subtle dysfunction in the communication from taste sensors to the brain and intestines. In other words, the experience of intense sweetness in the mouth appears to trigger a metabolic response that prepares the body for an enormous carbohydrate load. When those calories are not delivered, the body is still "primed," and it may be that subsequent calories are more likely to be stored as fat.

There is also a psychological theory as to why diet soft drink users end up gaining weight. By consuming low-calorie beverages, they may feel that they've been so virtuous that they reward themselves later with a second helping of lasagna.

All this research is provocative but not conclusive. Of course, one salient point is not debatable. Since the advent of artificial sweeteners and diet foods the prevalence of obesity in this country has dramatically *increased*, not decreased.

CONCLUSION

The DHEA Plan makes weight loss easier by helping to correct the underlying metabolic defects that cause cravings, fatigue, and other obstacles. DHEA appears to decrease the conversion of glucose to fat. What's more, maintaining prime peak levels of DHEA and bioenergetic nutrients can "tune up" your metabolism, making exercise easier and more enjoyable. I've presented a number of hints and given you numerous tools to improve your chance of success, but weight management is still a difficult endeavor.

Losing weight is a complex process that involves physical, mental, and social systems. Eating habits are by far the most difficult habits to change or break, primarily because we can never go "cold turkey." Food is always with us, and eating is a requirement for living. Every day we have to make decisions about which foods we're going to eat and which foods we aren't going to eat.

Rather than going on any kind of forced, controlled program, I encourage you to relearn what it takes to keep your body healthy and energetic. As you improve your metabolism and increase your activity level, you will move toward a balance that will keep you at an ideal weight for your body structure.

However, there are also some mental tips that can help you achieve permanent weight loss. The first is to start listening to your body. Rather than thinking about how your body looks and measuring your progress by the scale or tape measure, try to be aware of how your body *feels*. Your body wants to feel healthy and energetic. For it to feel active and vital, it needs to be nourished with good food, pure water, and clean air.

As you start to listen to your body, you'll know when it's hungry and what kind of food it needs to feel healthy. If you're listening to your body, you won't "eat by the clock" but will eat when you're hungry. If you're listening to your body, you will naturally stop eating when it is satisfied. With conventional diets that involve deprivation, the noise level created by the various food cravings you're experiencing makes it almost impossible to listen carefully to your body.

PUT A HALT TO EATING TRIGGERS

The second tip is to understand what triggers eating. Food is an integral part of our social life, a way we interact with each other, a way we reward ourselves, and a way we console ourselves. There are thousands of social and emotional cues that trigger eating, and they probably will never change. What can change, however, is our awareness of eating triggers and the choices we make in responding to them.

One popular acronym that helps us remember the primary eating triggers is HALT: hungry, angry, lonely, tired. These are the big four, followed closely by boredom/depression. We will never be able to completely remove these feelings from our lives, but we can choose positive ways to respond to them.

Here are just a few alternatives to eating triggers:

HUNGRY. The first thing to remember is, *if you're hungry, eat.* However, if you aren't sure you're feeling real hunger, here are two major things you can do to check: Take an activity break or drink a glass of water. Sometimes the hunger will go away.

ANGRY. Express your anger: write a letter even if you tear it up later, hit a pillow, go off by yourself and yell and scream. Work it off: take a brisk walk, sweep the sidewalk, clean the kitchen, wash the car.

LONELY. Reach out to someone: write a letter, make a phone call, volunteer your services. Pamper yourself: get a haircut, have a massage, take a yoga class, soak in a hot tub.

TIRED. Take an activity break: work in the garden, do some stretching, ride a bike. Feed your soul: arrange some flowers, walk through a beautiful park, listen to relaxing music.

BORED. Do something new: go to a museum, attend a lecture, introduce yourself to a neighbor. Learn something new: take a class, identify all the trees and flowers in your neighborhood, study ancient hieroglyphs. Contribute something: volunteer time at a local school, make soup for the homeless, visit a shut-in.

ONE LAST LOOK

I am always intrigued by the Paleolithic perspective, especially when it comes to the quality of life. We know from looking at hunters and gatherers today that they have more leisure time than do most middle-class Americans. What's more, they are relatively free of the diseases that kill 75 percent of us. Cancer is rare; heart disease and diabetes are unknown to people who live in harmony with their habitat. I have only visited one such tribe, but I was struck most by their energy, enthusiasm, and joy. Life for them is filled with adventure.

Of course, they are dwindling in number and soon will be gone. There is just no more wild space. But their faces keep coming back to me, along with their lithe, muscular bodies. They don't worry about their weight, and much of this chapter was developed from lessons I learned from them. Eat slowly and frequently. Eat foods as close as possible to the natural state. Exercise regularly and with a wide range of motion. Eat only when hungry and stop when the hunger is gone. These are all valuable tips, but there's one more very important ingredient to this awareness. I call it the power of passion.

There is something very special about having a zest for life. It seems that everything else falls into place when we're on fire with a new idea, a commitment, a career, our family, or life in general. I believe that the conveniences of modern life are a mixed blessing. They enable us to live in comfort, but that comfort often comes at the price of apathy and illness. If maintaining comfort, for example, requires us to spend each day doing a job that we hate, that's a bad bargain. If the comforts you provide merely allow your children to become obese at an early age, that's the opposite of progress—it's destruction.

I want to encourage you to break out. I believe we all need to express ourselves in unique and constructive ways. It may be music or art, drama or sports. You may choose a dozen different outlets in the course of a lifetime; just don't stop learning and growing. Don't stop moving, either. If your expression, activity, or new skills help someone else, all the better. Service to others provides rewards that no self-centered action can achieve. It taps into levels of energy and vitality you may never have experienced before. The DHEA Plan can provide the raw materials and information, but your own motivation and passion are the most important keys to success in weight management—and in life as a whole.

BIBLIOGRAPHY

Bates GW Jr., Egerman RS, Umstot ES, Buster JE, Casson PR. Dehydroepiandrosterone attenuates study-induced declines in insulin sensitivity in postmenopausal women. *Ann NY Acad Sci* 1995; 774:291–3.

Blundell JE, Hill AJ. Paradoxical effects of an intense sweetener (aspartame) on appetite. *Lancet* 1986; 1:1092–3.

Buffington CK, Pourmotabbed G, Kitabchi AE. Case report: Amelioration of insulin resistance in diabetes with dehydroepiandrosterone. *Am J Med Sci* 1993; 306:320–4.

Denke MA, Sempos CT, Grundy SM. Excess body weight: An under-recognized contributor to dyslipidemia in white American women. *Arch Intern Med* 1994; 154(4):401–10.

Fabry PJ, Fodor J, Hejl Z, Braun T, Zvolankova K. The frequency of meals: Its relationship to overweight, hypercholesterolemia, and decreased glucose tolerance. *Lancet* 1964; 2:614.

Hollifield G, Parson W. Metabolic adaptations to a "stuff and starve" feeding program: I. Studies of adipose tissue and liver glycogen in rats limited to a short daily feeding period. *J Clin Investi* 1962; 41:245.

Manson JE, Colditz GA, Stampfer MJ, Willett WC, Rosner B, Monson RR, Speizer FE, Hennekens CH. A prospective study of obesity and risk of coronary heart disease in women. *N Engl J Med* 1990; 322(13):882–9.

Schwartz AG, Hard GC, Pashko LL, Abou-Gharbia M, Swern D. Dehydroepiandrosterone: An antiobesity and anti-carcinogenic agent. *Nutri Cancer* 1981; 3:46–53.

Schwartz B. *Diets Don't Work*. Breakthru Publishing, Houston, 1982.

Stellman S, Garfinkel L. Short report: Artificial sweetener use and weight changes among women. *Prev Med*, 1986; 15:195–202.

Svec F, Porter Jr. Synergistic anorectic effect of DHEA and fenfluramine on Zucker rat food intake and selection: The obesity research program. *Ann NY Acad Sci* 1995; 774:332–4.

Svendsen OL, Hassager C, Christiansen C. Effect of an energy-restrictive diet, with or without exercise, on lean tissue mass, resting metabolic rate, cardiovascular risk factors, and bone in overweight postmenopausal women. *Am J Med* 1993: 95(2): 131–40.

Tepperman J. Gluconeogenesis, lipogenesis, and the Sherringtonian metaphor. *Fed Proc* 1970; 29:1281.

Yen SS, Morales AJ, Khorram O. Replacement of DHEA in aging men and women. *Ann NY Acad Sci* 1995; 774:128–42.

Yen TT, Allan JA, Pearson DV, Acton JM, Greenberg MM. Prevention of obesity in Avy/a mice by dehydroepiandrosterone. *Lipids* 1977; 12:409–13.

CHAPTER 9

Nutrition and the DHEA Plan: How to Eat Like a Cave Person

Good nutrition provides the foundation of your success with the DHEA Plan. In fact, the U.S. surgeon general has stated that if you do not drink excessively or smoke cigarettes, the single most important factor influencing your health (and therefore how long you live) is nutrition. Studies show that three of five hospital admissions could be avoided if people had better diets and lifestyle habits.

These are just facts and figures. To make them real, you might want to take a trip to your local hospital. Walk through the wards and ask how many people are looking forward to their treatments. We spend roughly 94 cents out of every health care dollar on treatment and practically nothing on prevention. But when it comes right down to it, there isn't a single person who wouldn't rather have prevented his or her problem.

How did we get into such a mess? I believe it is because there is no fresh air, whole grain, exercise, broccoli, or carrot lobby. All our attention is focused on treatment because that's where the money is. Health care today is like a city fire department with the latest high-tech equipment. Every time the city increases the budget, the fire department buys more equipment and continues to neglect fire prevention measures. This appears to be a fabulous fire department, because every time there's a fire, it races to the scene with the fancy equipment. It's exciting and very impressive, only pretty soon people start to notice that every year there are more fires.

You can look at health statistics and see the same scenario.

Cancer is increasing, and so are diabetes, autoimmune diseases, and obesity. Mortality from heart disease has finally started to fall, but even there the improvement is due primarily to diet and lifestyle changes. We as a society need to look at the path we're on and ask ourselves if it's where we really want to go. I think it's time to put more attention and resources into prevention, and nutrition is the key. Every cell in your body, from the top of your head to the tip of your toes, is manufactured from the food you eat. One of the most obvious points to be made about health is that wellness depends on optimum nutrition.

AN UNDERNOURISHED NATION

Government surveys and independent studies point out that the quality of the standard American diet has been decreasing steadily for over four decades. In 1955 Health, Education, and Welfare investigators estimated that 62 percent of the people surveyed had an adequate diet. By 1965, using the same criteria, that figure was down to 50 percent, and in 1989 it was 47 percent.

Analysis of a USDA food consumption survey reveals that *none* of the twenty thousand people studied consumed 100 percent of the RDA for all major nutrients. Interestingly, this does not appear to be an economic issue. Even people who can afford excellent food often end up with inadequate vitamin and mineral intake because of poor food selection. Today, *nearly 40 percent* of the average American diet consists of empty calories from sugar, desserts, fats, beverages, and snacks.

Equally important is the issue of *quantity*. Studies show that even with careful planning, a man needs to consume about 2,000 calories and a woman about 1,500 calories to obtain adequate amounts of vitamins and minerals. On the basis of this fact alone we can assume that 90 million Americans who are on low-calorie weight-loss diets are malnourished to a significant degree.

As we grow older, of course, things get worse. A number of factors contribute to decreased nutrition intake and absorption. Physicians are finally beginning to refer patients to trained nutritionists. These health professionals, using food intake diaries and computer analyses, can evaluate their clients' nutritional status and make recommendations for proper food selection and the prudent use of nutritional supplements.

Even the best diet, however, does not guarantee optimum nutrition. The all-important factors of digestion and metabolism must also be considered. Conditions that significantly decrease nutrient absorption include pancreatic, gallbladder, and liver disorders; food allergies; irritation and inflammation of the intestine or colon; surgery on the digestive tract; insufficient acid production in the stomach; low enzyme production; antibiotic therapy; lack of exercise; chronic use of antacids and laxatives; protein deficiency; yeast overgrowth; parasitic infections; and physical or emotional stress.

Even the common habits of eating fast and not chewing food well can cause decreased nutrient absorption. In addition to treating the above conditions and eating slowly and chewing well, you may want to consider the use of nutritional supplements as "insurance" against suboptimal absorption. It's important to realize that supplements are meant not to *substitute* for a proper diet but to augment the diet and in some cases improve the digestion, absorption, and metabolism of vital nutrients.

REFINED IS ROBBED BLIND

If you're like most Americans, the majority of your diet consists of refined and processed foods. Refining and processing remove important nutrients. The processing of wheat into white flour, for example, eliminates 85 percent of the coenzyme Q, 90 percent of the vitamin E, and virtually all of the fiber. The fact that manufacturers then "enrich" white flour with thiamine, riboflavin, and niacin is a joke, since they previously removed or reduced nineteen vitamins and minerals!

By eating a highly processed diet you run the risk of being undernourished no matter how much food you eat, and no vitamin pill can make up for that. I believe there are factors in whole natural foods that have not even been identified. A new mineral was discovered in 1995.

What do I mean by natural foods? Primarily fresh fruits and vegetables, whole grains, beans, eggs, and moderate amounts of animal protein—fish, chicken, and red meat. What I *don't* mean is any foods that didn't exist ten thousand years ago, including high-sugar, high-fat items such as candy, soft drinks, potato chips, popcorn, and ice cream.

You may ask, Why would I want to eat like a cave person? I thought you'd never ask.

OUR PAST AS HUNTER-GATHERERS

For most of the past 1.6 million years humans lived as hunters and gatherers. We inhabited jungles and dense forests where food was plentiful. Whenever we were hungry, we could pick fruit off a tree or dig up a root and eat it. When tasty animals such as deer or bison passed through, we would kill and eat them to supplement our daily diet of plant foods. When the food supply wore thin, we picked up and moved to a better place.

Even by modern standards our hunter-gatherer ancestors were incredibly fit, vibrant individuals. All the foods they consumed were unadulterated and unprocessed, so their energy levels stayed naturally high. Plus, for every 2,500 calories gathered, nearly 1,000 were expended, producing lean bodies with "all muscle and no fat."

Contrary to popular belief, our Paleolithic ancestors were not stubby, chimplike creatures; they stood almost as tall as we do today. Paleopathologists have determined that the height of hunter-gatherers around the end of the last ice age was five feet nine inches for men and five feet five inches for women. In fact, our ancestors' height actually *decreased* with the advent of agriculture, a point we'll revisit later in this chapter.

OUR GENETIC LEGACY

Even though over a million years of human evolution has come and gone, our genetic makeup is essentially the same as that of our Paleolithic forebears. Our DNA has not changed in twenty thousand years. And only in the past two hundred years has Western civilization spawned sedentary individuals who gobble foods high in sugar, salt, and saturated fats, a development that may prove to be our downfall.

You see, our genes did not prepare us for the diet-related health problems that plague us today. Some researchers believe that by returning to Paleolithic diet and exercise patterns, we can put an end to the diseases of civilization, including atherosclerosis, osteoporosis, hypertension, diabetes, and some cancers. These diseases are virtually unknown in the world's remaining hunter-gatherer societies.

Are we afflicted with "diseases of civilization" simply because we live longer? It's a common argument, but little evidence exists to support it. On the contrary, degenerative diseases can be found in the early stages among the children of Western societies, a phenomenon that is not present in hunter-gatherer cultures. In addition, primitive men and women who reach age sixty or more usually remain free of such disorders for the rest of their lives. That's a striking contrast to America, where the elderly are typically afflicted by at least one, if not several, degenerative diseases.

Paleolithic people had to contend with physical dangers that kept their life spans shorter than ours. We would never willingly face those perils today, and fortunately, we don't have to. But on a nutritional level they were head and shoulders above us. Since we share the same genes, there's much to learn from our ancestors' approach to nutrition.

THE IMPORTANCE OF A VARIED DIET

Surprisingly, our hunter-gatherer ancestors ate a wider variety of foods than do most modern men and women. This is true even of the fifty or so remaining hunter-gatherer groups on the planet. For example, the Kalahari Bushmen of Africa eat around seventy-five different wild plants. It's highly unlikely that they would ever die of starvation as the Irish did in the potato famine of the 1840s.

Variety is one of the most important principles of optimum nutrition because whatever nourishment you don't get from one food, you can get from another. In America we have plenty of food choices but not much variety. Surveys show that the average educated American eats no more than eleven types of food.

How can that be possible? Everyone insists that we have a more varied diet. But when you ask about grains, for example, a typical list includes bread, rolls, breakfast cereal, crackers, cookies, sandwiches, spaghetti, pasta, cakes, and biscotti—all of which are simply different forms of wheat.

You get the idea. We tend to eat what our mothers prepared. We eat what we like. We get into food ruts that last until our awareness changes and we realize that we live on a planet with incredible diversity. There's a reason for diversity. It's not just for show. If we choose it, a varied diet assures that we will be optimally nourished for a long and healthy lifetime.

THINK LIKE A CAVE PERSON

There are scores of nutrition books that make the simple act of eating an extremely complex matter, but good nutrition is not rocket science. All you have to do is think like a cave person. What did they eat, and how did they eat it?

Did cave people have microwaves? Did they eat plasticized fats called margarine or refined carbohydrates called Gummi bears? Did they drink shots of 100-proof alcohol? Of course not. Neither was their food grown in depleted soil, harvested before it was ripe, or transported thousands of miles and stored for months or years.

The more you can imitate a cave person's lifestyle, the better your health will be. Remember the evolutionary timeline that stretches the length of a football field? Modern food choices represent less than 1 inch. Our bodies haven't had time to adapt to processed foods. Eating them throws our metabolism into a state of confusion from which we are practically helpless to recover. That brings us to an important question regarding agriculture.

WAS AGRICULTURE A MISTAKE?

A group of highly respected scientists believes that agriculture was the downfall of the human race. As unusual as this viewpoint is, it has some merit for the investigation at hand.

The advent of agriculture about ten thousand years ago profoundly changed the course of human history. From that point until the present the agricultural revolution has gradually taken over the planet. Very few tribes of hunters and gatherers remain. Of course, we've been taught that agriculture was a boon to humankind. The party line goes that agriculture enabled humans to stay in one place and raise more food with less work. But did it really happen that way? Studies of present-day Bushmen show that they work far less than do their neighbors who raise crops. In addition, their hunting and gathering lifestyle gives the Bushmen more leisure and more time to sleep.

Examples abound from other regions as well. Anthropologists have found that some hunter-gatherers actually became shorter after the introduction of agriculture, a fate from which their descendants have not fully recovered. Another study of Indian skeletons found in the Illinois River Valley showed a major health decline after maize farming began around A.D. 1150.

Driven by the demands of an increasing population, many primitive peoples adopted farming from necessity rather than by choice. In the process, quality was traded for quantity in their diets. There's no doubt that farming can support more people per square mile than hunting and gathering can, but where does that leave us today? We're down to three crops—wheat, rice, and corn—that provide most of the calories consumed by humans. And each one of the three is lacking in certain vitamins and amino acids that are necessary for good health.

It's not realistic to expect one or two or even three foods to supply complete nutrition, but there's no turning back. We're not about to reject agriculture and the foods it produces. But the point is to try to emulate the hunter-gatherers and vary your diet. If you eat seventy-five varieties of plants as the Bushmen do, there's no doubt your health will be the better for it.

THE GRAZING LIFESTYLE

As was mentioned above, studies of present-day hunter-gatherers show that they have much more leisure time than "civilized" people do. That may seem surprising, but when you don't eat much, you don't have to spend much time working (searching for food). Hunter-gatherers know that it takes a small quantity of food to satisfy hunger. If you don't believe this, try it yourself. Next time you're hungry, be sensitive to the point when your hunger is gone. Most people find it's somewhere between one-third and one-half of the meal.

We civilized folks eat beyond the point where our hunger ends because we know the next meal is four to five hours (or more) away. Hunter-gatherers don't operate on this schedule. They will eat again in an hour if they get hungry. The hunter-gatherer style of eating, known as *grazing*, is without a doubt the most efficient way to eat.

Studies show that people who consume 2,000 calories a day by grazing tend to lose weight, while people eating the same number of calories at lunch and dinner (as 90 percent of Americans do) tend to gain weight.

GRAZING IN THE 1990s

You can get in the habit of grazing by keeping healthful snacks in the office and the house. Fresh vegetables and fruit are the best choices, followed by whole grain crackers, rice cakes, and other high-fiber grain products.

Every couple of hours munch on one of your healthy snacks. When lunchtime rolls around, you'll find your appetite much subdued. Repeat the same thing in the afternoon and you'll find that you won't be staking so much importance on dinner. You'll find it easy to consume smaller portions at meals because your body's energy needs will have been satisfied consistently throughout the day. Your blood sugar levels will be stabilized, and as a result your energy level will stay consistently high rather than swinging wildly up and down.

OMNIVOROUS-R-US

For over a million years our ancestors' survival depended on plant foods. Fruits and vegetables had the advantage of not running or swimming away. However, that doesn't mean we're naturally vegetarians—far from it! The reason *Homo sapiens* evolved is largely a matter of our status as omnivores. Humans have always possessed the ability to eat a wide variety of foods of both plant and animal origin. In Paleolithic times, our far-ranging diet choices did much to ensure the survival of the species.

Today our diet choices are even more diverse and some might say downright destructive. To the abundant offerings of Mother Nature we've added thousands of refined and processed foods with a nutritional value ranging from marginal to zero. (Marshmallows, which consist entirely of food additives and not one gram of real food, win the booby prize.)

KEY FACTORS IN THE PALEOLITHIC DIET

In the Paleolithic diet 60 percent of the daily calories come from complex carbohydrates such as fruits, vegetables, and whole grains. Fats and proteins contribute 20 to 25 percent each. See the chart below for a list of preferred foods and follow the accompanying principles for the best results:

PALEOLITHIC DIET PREFERRED FOODS

Fresh vegetables and fruits: five servings per day
Whole grains, beans, and cereals: five servings per day
Dairy products (milk, cheese, etc.): one serving per day
Meat, eggs, chicken, and fish: two servings per day
Water: eight glasses per day

- Eat as many foods as possible in their raw natural state.
- Avoid refined and processed foods of any kind.
- Limit servings of animal fat and full-fat dairy products.
- Obtain quality protein from meats not treated with additives or hormones as well as fresh or frozen fish.

WHAT ABOUT THE FOUR BASIC FOOD GROUPS?

In the true Paleolithic diet of our ancestors the four basic food groups were really the two basic food groups. The ancients had meat and fish as the first group and vegetables and fruits as the second. They consumed neither dairy products nor breads and cereals, which we know as the third and fourth food groups.

However, in adapting the Paleolithic diet for modern use, we found it impossible to completely eliminate these foods because we've come to depend on them so much. We recommend eating breads and cereals that are high in fiber and limiting consumption of dairy products to one serving per day. The high level of fat in dairy products is what you're trying to avoid.

PEAS, GLORIOUS PEAS

There's a wonder food waiting for you in the freezer section of your grocery store: frozen peas. Frozen green peas are picked and packaged so fast that they have virtually the same nutrition value as fresh peas. A three-quarter-cup serving contains 6 grams of protein, less than 1 gram of fat, 3.5 grams of fiber, and 35 mg of calcium. *Lunchbox tip:* If you pack a salad, top it off with frozen peas. They will thaw by lunchtime and keep your salad fresh and cold in the process.

WHEN IN DOUBT, EAT VEGETABLES

Vegetables are a cornucopia of vitamins, minerals, essential fats, complex carbohydrates, and even protein. You can't go wrong eating vegetables. So much nutrition is packed into vegetables that you could live on nothing else for a considerable length of time.

Variety is the spice of life, and so it is with vegetables. Don't limit your choices to carrot and celery sticks or a few broccoli florets. Most supermarkets have over fifty kinds of vegetables to choose from, and you can eat them broiled, barbecued, steamed, sauteed, or raw. High in fiber and low in calories, vegetables form the foundation of a healthy Paleolithic diet.

FAT, FAT, AND MORE FAT

Thousands of years ago our ancestors ate wild game whenever they could, and so do hunter-gatherers today. The difference in fat content between this wild meat and domesticated beef is staggering. A study of fifteen species of African herbivores showed a carcass fat content of just 3.9 percent. In contrast, thanks to modern breeding and feeding practices, beef carcasses contain 25 to 35 percent fat.

Not only is our meat marbled with fat, fat confronts us everywhere we turn—from salads laced with dressing, to baked potatoes smothered with sour cream, to mountains of smooth, frosty ice cream. No wonder it's so easy to obtain 40 percent of our calories from fat, as most Americans do. These fats choke our arteries and add significantly to the risk of stroke and heart disease.

The Paleolithic diet calls for limiting dairy products for this reason. While meats are valuable sources of protein, we recommend lean meats raised without hormones, free-range chickens, and fresh or frozen fish whenever possible.

THE EXERCISE FACTOR

Since hunter-gatherers spent much of their time on the move finding food, it's no surprise that the most important nonfood factor in the Paleolithic diet is exercise. Your goal should be to generate enough exercise, in addition to your normal activity, to burn about 2,000 calories per week. See Chapter 7 for recommendations on developing an exercise program that works for you.

Every calorie you ingest has a fate, a destination somewhere in the body, and that destination depends on the dialogue between your stomach, your brain, and your muscles. For the dialogue you want to hear, you need an active body. Unfortunately, the modern-day dialogue goes something like this:

STOMACH: We just took in 800 calories, Boss, what do you want us to do with them?

BRAIN: I don't know. Let me ask the muscles. Muscles, do you need any energy?

MUSCLES: No, Boss. We didn't move all day.

BRAIN: Okay. Stomach, let's convert all those calories to fat.

The Paleolithic version of this dialogue is much different. For starters, only 300 to 500 calories are consumed at one time instead of 800 to 1,000. Then, when the brain checks in with the muscles, they say, "Boy, we've been working hard. Send us as much energy as you can." As a result, all the available calories are sent to the muscles (or stored in the liver as energy) and none are stored as fat.

DISEASE PREVENTION AND THE PALEOLITHIC DIET

The Paleolithic diet has specific benefits that help you fight the most common diseases of civilization, as follows:

• **CANCER**. Scientists recently identified a new nutrient group known as *phytochemicals*, which appear to turn on anticancer enzymes in your cells. These substances occur naturally in fruits and vegetables such as garlic, cruciferous vegetables, and citrus fruits, all of which have played an important role in cancer prevention research and all of which are important in the Paleolithic diet.

• **DIABETES**. Because you stabilize your blood sugar levels by grazing throughout the day rather than eating two or three large meals, you greatly decrease the risk of developing diabetes as an adult.

• **ATHEROSCLEROSIS**. By limiting your fat intake to 25 grams or less per day, you decrease the risk of artery blockage and heart disease.

• **OSTEOPOROSIS**. Eating generous quantities of fresh vegetables and fruits optimizes your mineral intake. When you add the exercise factor and supplements described in Chapter 6, you can develop stronger bones and lessen the chance of bone fractures.

• **HYPERTENSION**. Exercise and a natural foods diet can dramatically reduce the incidence of hypertension (high blood pressure). A natural foods diet is low in sodium and high in potassium and calcium, substances that help keep blood pressure low. Exercise lowers blood pressure and helps reduce stress.

LONGEVITY AND THE PALEOLITHIC DIET

Aside from the fact that avoiding diseases will enable you to live longer, there appears to be a positive longevity factor in the Paleolithic diet. Researchers have not been able to explain it fully, but when animals are given fewer calories, they live longer, sometimes 30 to 50 percent longer than their fed-to-the-max peers. This has been documented in a number of primates.

Recently, a group of investigators tested the theory that DHEA might be involved. Sure enough, calorie restriction led to significant increases in DHEA in rhesus monkeys, possibly as a result of a de-

---

BEST EATING PRACTICES

- Eat only when you are hungry.
- Eat sitting down in a calm environment (this does not include the car).
- Eat without distractions (distractions include radio, television, newspapers, books, and intense or anxiety-producing conversations).
- Eat until your hunger is satisfied and then stop, knowing that you can eat again later if you're hungry.
- Eat slowly and chew each mouthful.
- Eat with enjoyment, pleasure, and gusto.
- Use an important twentieth-century advantage—nutritional supplementation. Maintain prime peak levels of DHEA, optimal bioenergetic nutrition, antioxidants, and nutritional support for bones, tendons, ligaments, and joints.

---

crease in insulin levels. Longevity experts have long advocated what Dr. Roy Walford calls a "high nutrient, low calorie diet," and many are now looking at the added benefit of keeping DHEA at prime peak.

GO MEDITERRANEAN

If the idea of a Paleolithic diet leaves you cold, a Mediterranean-style diet is an excellent substitute. The emphasis is on fresh vegetables, fruits, and whole grains, with moderate amounts of fish, chicken, and red meat. Other components of the Mediterranean diet include heart-healthy and immune-stimulating items such as olive oil (which actually helps lower serum cholesterol), garlic (which decreases platelet aggregation and lowers blood pressure), tomatoes and tomato sauce (which contain high levels of lycopene, a potent anticancer carotenoid), and wine (which can decrease abnormal clot formation when used in moderation).

No one knows what ingredients are most responsible for their

excellent health, but surveys show that some Mediterranean people enjoy protection against heart disease equal to or better than that of American vegetarians. Mediterranean people are also very social, and studies show that community builds immunity. The region's legendary sunshine also makes an important contribution to overall health and well-being.

The Mediterranean diet can provide an easy transition between a diet of highly processed foods and the Paleolithic diet. As in all things, the key is moderation. Stick to one glass of wine per day and go easy on the pasta. Above all, remember that eating is one of the great pleasures in life.

DIGESTION: IS WHAT YOU EAT WHAT YOU GET?

When it comes to food, we suffer from a number of false perceptions. One of the most pervasive and dangerous misconceptions in nutrition is the idea that "what you eat is what you get." We forget that food, once swallowed, is still technically "outside" the body (much as the hole is outside the doughnut) until it is digested and absorbed through the intestinal tract into the bloodstream. The misconception is that this occurs easily, that by some automatic process everything we eat is broken down and absorbed and that the remaining undigested fiber is eliminated as waste.

In reality, the digestive process is neither easy nor automatic. It is an intricate and continuous process with numerous mechanical and chemical reactions taking place simultaneously. Furthermore, each step in the process is dependent on other steps, and a defect in one phase will almost certainly hinder the entire process to some degree. This critical function, by which we are nourished and thrive, deserves close attention. For a biochemist, digestion requires diligent research into the science of acid, enzyme, and hormone release. For the individual, it means learning the signs of maldigestion and the methods one can employ to improve this vital function.

"I CAN'T BELIEVE I ATE THE WHOLE THING"

For many people the signs of maldigestion are apparent only when

abdominal pain or heartburn sends us running to the medicine cabinet. The problem is that these painful conditions are the end result of a long chain of chemical events stemming from putrefaction and fermentation. The use of antacids and plop-fizz remedies is clearly closing the barn door long after the horse is gone. We must look for the cause of the problem, not just treat the symptoms. In fact, chronic use of these common remedies can cause significant harm.

To discover the cause of maldigestion, we need to learn about the process of normal digestion, and how that process is impaired.

Phase I: "The thought of food makes my mouth water."

Have you ever wondered how that happens? It's the result of what is called the *cephalic* phase of digestion. Digestion actually begins before you put food in your mouth. The sight, smell, or even thought of food puts the digestive process in gear. Salivary enzymes are secreted in the mouth, and hydrochloric acid secretion prepares the stomach to work on the food once it's swallowed. For this reason, one should try to relax before eating. Don't rush; enjoy the anticipation of a nourishing meal.

Unfortunately, we often see the opposite: Drive-through fast-food restaurants, for example, promote "freeway lunches" in which the major thought is not the enjoyment of the food but how to keep from spilling your thick shake in stop-and-go traffic. In the same way anxiety and stress before a meal impair this phase of digestion, and almost everyone has experienced the consequences of feeling later as if one had eaten rocks for lunch.

Phase II: The first mouthful

Our saliva contains a very important digestive enzyme called amylase and a group of antibodies called secretory immunoglobulin A (IgA). The amylase initiates starch digestion, and the IgA fights bacteria in the oral cavity. Since the effectiveness of both substances depends on adequate contact with food, one can easily improve phase II digestion by chewing well and eating slowly. Studies have shown that it's not so much the presence of food in your mouth that starts the digestive enzymes flowing but the actual action of the jaws in chewing the food.

Phase III: Acids and enzymes

By this point the stomach should be well prepared to deal with ingested food. Hydrochloric acid (HCL) secretion by the stomach began with the mental anticipation of eating and was further stimulated by the mechanical action of chewing. Dietary protein causes the release of a hormone in the stomach called gastrin, which stimulates further secretion of HCL. Adequate HCL secretion is essential for every phase of digestion from this point on. For example, the enzyme pepsin, which is also secreted by the stomach, has little effect on food unless the contents of the stomach are acidified by adequate HCL. In addition, HCL is a vital bactericidal agent that protects us from dangerous disease-causing agents. Finally, it is the acidity of the food passing from the stomach into the small intestine that causes the pancreas to secrete digestive enzymes and bicarbonate, which are essential for phase IV digestion.

What has occurred in the stomach is breakdown. Almost all absorption takes place in the small intestine, but the stomach's job of mixing enzymes and acid is of the utmost importance. Inadequate HCL secretion is therefore a real problem and is commonly caused by a number of factors. Insufficient dietary protein, though not common in America, can impair gastrin secretion and thus decrease HCL production. As we mentioned earlier, eating too fast or in a state of anxiety can also decrease HCL. Finally and most important, research has shown that as we grow older, our production of HCL often decreases dramatically.

Phase IV: Absorption (maybe)

If all goes well, the final phase of digestion is accomplished primarily in the small intestine, where the pancreas, liver, gallbladder, and intestinal lining provide enzymes and other biochemicals that act on the food. The breakdown of food is completed, and absorption takes place. If only it were that simple. Here is the heart of the misconception: The fats are neatly broken down into fatty acids, the carbohydrates become simple sugars, and the proteins are reduced completely to amino acids. The fact is that this process occurs with varying degrees of efficiency, depending on the multitude of factors we've discussed.

If, for example, pancreatic enzyme secretion was inadequate, none of the above reactions are completed satisfactorily—and that's just one possible scenario. Four major problems result from maldigestion:

1. Malnutrition. If foods are not properly broken down, the constituent vitamins, minerals, and proteins are not absorbed.

2. Food allergy. Recent research has shown conclusively that small amounts of incompletely digested protein are absorbed through the intestinal wall into the bloodstream. Obviously, the body is going to react to the presence of these foreign particles in the blood, and a full-scale allergy reaction may follow. Since the problem factor is now circulating in the bloodstream, allergic symptoms can and do occur anywhere in the body. Joints and muscles may be inflamed or painful, and brain biochemistry may be altered to produce headache, depression, confusion, anxiety, or behavioral disorders.

3. Proper digestion is necessary for the secretion of CCK, which is primarily responsible for turning off the appetite. CCK production is especially impaired when a meal is consumed rapidly. Thus, a fast eater not only impairs digestion but often adds insult to injury by overeating.

4. The last unfortunate consequence of maldigestion involves what eventually *happens* to all that undigested and unabsorbed food. Keep in mind that it's quite warm (98.6°F) and very moist in the intestines. As this food passes into the colon, the conditions are perfect for fermentation. Bacteria that are naturally present in the colon cause carbohydrates to ferment and proteins to putrefy. Aside from the uncomfortable gas and bloating that result, fermentation and putrefaction lead to the production of toxic waste materials that can be absorbed into the body.

Researchers are beginning to look at this as a serious problem that increases in severity the longer maldigestion is allowed to continue. Ultimately, the barrier mechanism of the gastrointestinal tract may be compromised, allowing the passage of bacteria, toxins, and partially digested material directly into the bloodstream. This in turn sets off a full-scale immune response that generates significant and chronic metabolic stress.

We now know that metabolic stress contributes to the immune dysfunction that accompanies aging. While optimizing DHEA can help restore the balance, I believe it is extremely important to arrest the conditions that cause the problem. The take-home message here is that bad things happen when you don't digest your food completely.

SUMMARY

I've described four stages of digestion that begin with the mind and end with the action of bile and digestive enzymes in the small intestine. Let's now look at how you can analyze your digestive efficiency and what can be done to improve this vital function.

Begin by evaluating how you feel after a meal. Assuming that you did not overeat (in which case maldigestion is assured), you should experience no gas, bloating, or discomfort. In fact, except for the fact that you are no longer hungry, you should experience no significant change from how you felt before the meal.

Then look at your energy level. Many people assume that fatigue after a meal is normal, that somehow the digestive process requires so much energy that we need a nap to recover. This is not true at all. In fact, if anything, one should feel slightly energized after a meal. Fatigue is most often a sign of food allergy, maldigestion, or both. Next, look for signs of fermentation and putrefaction about an hour after eating, such as flatulence, bad breath, or foul-smelling stools.

STEPS TO BETTER DIGESTION

1. Eat like a hunter-gatherer.
   - Eat small amounts. The acid in your stomach is like a chemical fire that will burn efficiently if small branches are added a few at a time. Dumping huge logs on the fire will cause it to smolder and go out. Many experts today recommend four to five small meals rather than two or three large meals each day.
   - Chew your food well. Chewing well implies eating slowly, which is another aid to digestion. Remember that the premeal stomach is quite acidic, and the ingestion of food dilutes that acid. Effective digestion depends on the ability of the stomach to reacidify during a meal and to maintain a level of acid that

will activate gastric enzymes and initiate protein breakdown. It was believed that only the elderly suffer from insufficient stomach acid (hypochlorhydria), but extensive research has shown that the condition is common among individuals in all age groups.

- Eat foods as close as possible to their natural state. That means eating plenty of raw fruits and vegetables and whole grains and a minimum of refined and processed foods.

2. Don't wash your food down with a beverage, especially a soft drink. Your mother was right. Although beverages may provide the lubrication effect of saliva, they lack the amylase important for starch digestion. Contrary to popular belief, however, this does not mean we should avoid drinking water with meals. Studies show that 10 to 15 ounces of room-temperature water taken with a meal may enhance digestion. The point seems to be that the water and food should not be taken in the same mouthful and that the water should not be ice cold.

3. Last but not least is the essential factor of *relaxation*. Often we are rushed and anxious about eating or face difficult stress in our lives. Proper digestion requires a relaxed state of mind and body. Anxiety alters HCL production in the stomach and tightens abdominal muscles, interfering with normal peristaltic movement. Stress can make swallowing difficult and is a major factor in numerous eating disorders.

Classical or soft instrumental music tends to put people at ease when eating and results in a number of behavioral changes conducive to improved digestion. When volunteers were exposed to calming music, their pace of eating decreased dramatically, as did the size of the meals consumed. In fact, they took almost twice as long to eat fewer calories than they did when lively music was playing. They said that food tasted better and that they had fewer digestive complaints, plus a greater feeling of satisfaction from the meal. This makes perfect sense, as the longer we chew a food, the more pleasure we receive from the aroma (chewing forces air from the throat to the nose) and taste (starches are broken down into simple sugars by the salivary enzymes).

By contrast, jazz and rock music have been shown to increase eating speed and impair digestion. Volume also plays a significant role. Animal and human experiments show that as music volume is increased, there is a significant increase in meal size and the speed of eating.

FINAL HINTS

Once again the Paleolithic perspective gives us important hints about what and how to eat. If you follow these guidelines and still experience digestive problems, I recommend that you consult a doctor. Numerous disease states impair digestion, and you will want to rule them out. Your doctor may recommend an enzyme supplement which can do wonders, and if you are past age sixty, you may need that supplement for the rest of your life. It's a small price to pay for the benefits you'll receive. Remember that digestive efficiency decreases with age; there is a great deal to gain by restoring digestion to prime peak. In addition, effective stress revision is an indispensable ally in our quest for efficient digestion and optimum health.

THE MODERN ADVANTAGE: NUTRITIONAL SUPPLEMENTS

Perhaps the most significant nutritional advantage we have over our Paleolithic ancestors is the availability of vitamin and mineral supplements, which represent the fastest and most reliable way to improve our nutrition and overall health. As I have mentioned before, we must remember that the word *supplement* is literally the correct term. These products are meant to supplement a widely varied natural foods diet, not replace it. In this context, health experts generally agree that supplements can play an important role in a health and longevity program. If you need to be convinced, you will find a thoroughly researched presentation on the value of vitamin and mineral supplements in Appendix C.

For most people the question isn't "Should I take vitamins?" but "What should I take?" Popular magazines will give you wildly conflicting views, the wall of choices in the health food store will make your head spin, and your doctor will probably be of little help. But it's easier than you think.

GUIDELINES FOR CHOOSING NUTRITIONAL SUPPLEMENTS

Multiple Vitamins with Minerals

This is your foundation, your nutrition insurance, and the range of quality is enormous.

- Men and women have different nutritional needs. Look for a gender-specific multivitamin.
- There is no way you can put everything you need in one tablet, and even if you could, your body couldn't absorb it. Look for a multidose product that provides the full spectrum of nutrients in three to six tablets or capsules.
- Look for premium-quality ingredients. You can get minerals by eating dirt, but that's not very efficient. Many products include nutrient compounds that are not much better. Look for *chelated* minerals, or minerals bound to organic acids such as citric acid or aspartic acid. These citrates and aspartates have demonstrated superiority over common mineral salts.
- Avoid kitchen-sink formulas with forty or more ingredients. A good multivitamin should contain twenty-eight to thirty-two nutrients and need not provide dubious add-ons like bee pollen, algae, wheat grass, brewer's yeast, and mugwort.

Bioenergetics

These are your energy nutrients, and what you're looking for here are nonstimulant metabolic optimizers such as coenzyme Q10, alpha-ketoglutaric acid, chromium (I prefer the nicotinate compound), potassium and magnesium aspartate, and vitamin B_6. Useful add-ons include ginseng (in a standardized concentrate) and creatine, an energy buffer that provides fuel to the muscles in the late stages of exercise.

Bone, Joint, and Tendon Support

This should be comprehensive, including not only calcium but all the nutrients required for connective tissue health: magnesium, potassium, manganese, zinc, copper, boron, chromium, vitamin K, vitamin C, and vitamin D. Look for chondroitin sulfate or glucosamine sulfate (see Chapter 6) and premium calcium compounds such as hydroxyapatite and calcium citrate. Again, this should be in a multi-dose formulation for optimum absorption.

Extra Antioxidant Support

The thing to remember here is that different antioxidants protect the body in different ways. Therefore, look for a *comprehensive* product providing not only vitamins E, C, and beta-carotene but also bioflavonoids, niacinamide, folic acid, mixed carotenoids, and a group of important antioxidants known as proanthocyanidins, which are derived from pine bark or grape seeds.

A "Green Drink"

A variety of powders can be mixed in water or juice to make a concentrated nutrient beverage, or "green drink." Usually made from the immature grass of wheat, barley, or another grain, these products provide an extremely wide variety of known and potential nutrient factors.

Adaptogens

These are nutrients and herbs that are known to assist the body in dealing with stress. Some of them also enhance mental and physical performance, help lower blood pressure, enhance glucose metabolism, and accelerate enzyme systems that contribute to vitality and overall health.

We know that entire species of plants and animals are disappearing every day as the world's forests are cleared for industrial development, mining, logging, and livestock. No one knows the treasures that are being destroyed, but one thing is certain: The vast expanse of forest comprising more than 150,000 square miles along the Chinese/Russian border is among the most pristine and biologically diverse tracts of land on earth. And it is here that most adaptogenic herbs are to be found. Like green drinks and sea vegetables, it may be that adaptogens contain nutrients that formed a significant part of man's early diet, but which are absent in refined twentieth-century fare.

Look for Eleutherococcus (Siberian ginseng), Schizandra, and *Rhaponticum carthamoides*.

BIBLIOGRAPHY

Brewster L, Jacobson MF. *The Changing American Diet.* Center for Science in the Public Interest, Washington, D.C., 1978.

Crocetti and Guthrie. Eating behavior and associated nutrient quality of diets. Anarem Systems Research Corporation, October 1982.

Gibson RS, Scythes CA. Dietary chromium, selenium and other trace element intakes of a sample of Canadian pre-menopausal women. *Fed Proc* 1983; 42:816.

Greger JL, et al. Calcium, magnesium, phosphorus, copper and manganese balance in adolescent females. *Am J Clin Nutr* 1978; 31:117.

Hallfrisch J, Powell A, et al. Mineral balances of men and women consuming high fiber diets with complex or simple carbohydrate. *J Nutr* 1987; 117:48.

Kumpulainen JT, et al. Determination of chromium in selected United States diets. *J Agr Food Chem* 1979; 27:490.

Labuza R, Sloan T. *Food for Thought.* Avi, Westport, CT, 1976.

Lane MA, Ingram DK, Roth GS. Effects of aging and long-term calorie restriction on DHEA and DHEA sulfate in rhesus monkeys. *Ann NY Acad Sci* 1995; 774:319.

Lee CJ. Nutritional status of selected teenagers in Kentucky. *Am J Clin Nutr* 1978; 31:1453.

Mackie DA, Pangborn RM. Mastication and its influence on human salivary flow and alpha-amylase secretion. *Physiol Behav*, 1990; 47(3):593–5.

Nationwide Food Consumption Survey, 1977–1978. U.S. Dept. Agriculture, Science and Education Administration, Preliminary report No. 2, U.S. Government Printing Office, Washington, D.C., 1980.

Schwerin, HS, Stanton JL, Riley AM Jr, Brett BE. How have the quantity and quality of the American diet changed during the past decade? *Food Techn* 1981.

Tufts University Diet and Nutrition Letter 1991; 9(4)1–2.

Walford RL. *The 120 Year Diet.* Simon & Schuster, New York, 1986.

CHAPTER 10

The DHEA Story:
From Plant to Patient

For over twenty years DHEA for human use has been derived from plant compounds called *sapogenins*. The plants with the highest known concentrations of these substances are members of the Dioscoreaceae (yam) family. The story of the discovery of these plants is a fascinating one and ties in with the beginnings of hormone research around the turn of the century. This chapter delves into the history of DHEA production and discusses what you can expect today in terms of purity, potency, and truth in advertising.

A BRIEF HISTORY OF HORMONE PRODUCTION

The DHEA story dates back to 1905, when scientists first gave the name *hormones* to substances found in animal organs that they suspected could help human patients with deficiency diseases.

In the early 1920s several researchers and a handful of newly formed companies confirmed that hormones could have a dramatic effect on human physiology. In 1921 F. G. Banting and Charles H. Best of Toronto, Canada, isolated the first significant nonsteroidal hormone—insulin—a discovery that completely transformed the treatment of diabetes, which was then an incurable and often fatal disease. Banting and Best, along with Dr. J. J. R. MacLeod, received the Nobel Prize in 1923.

Encouraged by the success of insulin, other researchers studied estrogen, testosterone, cortisone, progesterone, and androsterone.

Also known as steroidal hormones, these were the most "popular" hormones studied during the 1920s, 1930s, and 1940s. But where was DHEA?

Researchers knew of DHEA's existence, but perhaps it didn't attract more attention because other hormones, such as testosterone, are far more potent, or "biologically active." A small amount of testosterone or insulin given to a laboratory animal would cause dramatic changes in metabolism and behavior, whereas small amounts of DHEA had no immediate effects. In the 1960s scientists would discover that DHEA is naturally present in our bodies in far greater amounts than is any other steroid hormone and that it can be converted to sex hormones on an as-needed basis.

In the 1970s they began to suspect that DHEA might have functions other than providing a "buffer" or reservoir for the sex hormones, and interest has been growing ever since. As a researcher recently put it, "DHEA doesn't just sit around waiting to be converted to something else. The problem is we don't have a clear picture of its full metabolic function." The bottom line is that DHEA has been clinically studied in humans for only the past ten to fifteen years, so the picture is still unfolding.

THE SEARCH FOR A SOURCE

In the 1930s and 1940s most steroidal hormones were extracted from animal organs. In those early days a huge number of animal organs were needed to make a very small amount of pure hormone. For example, one laboratory used the ovaries from fifty thousand sows to make 20 mg of pure progesterone.

Some hormones were made from animal cholesterol, which has the same "backbone" molecular structure as DHEA, testosterone, progesterone, and other hormones. But the output of hormones derived from cholesterol was small, and researchers were searching for a better raw material that could be of widespread commercial use.

In 1935 a chemist at the Rockefeller Institute, Russell E. Marker, believed he could find a new and better starting material for progesterone, the "pregnancy hormone." When the institute turned down his research proposal, he left for Pennsylvania State College with a fellowship supported by Parke, Davis & Co. He soon identified the source he was looking for—plant *sapogenins* (*sapo*, "soaplike")—the study of which occupied him for the remainder of his career.

Marker's studies resulted in the isolation and synthesis of a large number of new steroids, including DHEA. He published more than fifty scientific papers between 1935 and 1938, challenging other chemists regarding the structure of sapogenins and studying their chemical reactions to prove his findings. Perhaps his greatest commercial contribution was the "Marker degradation," a five-step chemical process still used to convert plant extracts to progesterone and other usable hormones—DHEA among them.

In 1936 other researchers isolated a sapogenin from a Japanese species of Dioscorea (the yam family) and named it diosgenin. Marker tested a sample of diosgenin with his Marker degradation and found that it was converted to progesterone and to other steroid hormones as well. Convinced that he had identified a cheap source material for the mass production of hormones, he then set off to find the best plant sources of diosgenin.

STALKING THE WILD DIOSCOREA

Marker arranged a series of botanical expeditions throughout the southern United States and Mexico, bringing back over four hundred species of plants for analysis. In 1943 he moved to Mexico, where he concentrated his search on two members of the Dioscoreaceae family, commonly known as the Mexican wild yam. The variety that turned out to be most valuable was *Dioscorea barbasco*.

Dioscorea species are tropical plants found in many parts of the world. They have a distinctive leaf with a small tail, and the vines emerge from a root that can be very large and bulbous.

For nearly three decades these plants were harvested in Mexico by foreign pharmaceutical companies on a commercial scale. As the demand grew, Mexican *yerberos* (medical plant vendors) had to travel deeper into the jungle to locate and harvest the plants. In response to this situation, the Mexican government began to restrict exports of diosgenin.

In 1975 the Mexican government prohibited new foreign companies from exploiting the plants for two reasons: to prevent extinction of the species and to allow the government to establish its own pharmaceutical hormone industry.

The government's effort failed, and most of the foreign pharmaceutical companies producing hormones chose to augment their supplies of diosgenin by going to other countries. The export of raw diosgenin from Mexico is still restricted.

Commercially available DHEA is now manufactured in a variety of places, most notably Europe and China. Aside from its current wave of popularity, DHEA is also important because pharmaceutical companies sometimes use it as a starting substance for manufacturing other steroid hormones.

NATURAL OR SYNTHETIC?

Most hormones produced in a "pure" form through large-scale commercial operations are prepared using both chemical and microbial (fermentation) processes, and DHEA is no exception.

There are numerous products on the market that claim to be "natural sources" of DHEA. Some people believe that taking a "natural" substance is better than taking a "synthetic" one, but consider this: Wild yams as such contain not DHEA but diosgenin, which is not natural to the human body. In fact, diosgenin may be *toxic* to humans. It must be converted through the Marker degradation to produce DHEA that the body can assimilate. *The human body cannot do this. It can be accomplished only in a laboratory.*

The reason is a chemical one. The structure of diosgenin has six carbon rings, while the sex hormones in our bodies, including DHEA, have four carbon rings. Two of diosgenin's rings must be broken to yield the four-ring human steroidal hormone structure before our bodies can use it as DHEA.

Thus, in the case of DHEA, what is "natural"? Diosgenin is natural to plants but not to humans. DHEA is natural to humans but not to plants. To get naturally occurring DHEA for supplementation, we need to partially synthesize it, starting with what Mother Nature has already built—the carbon ring structures of diosgenin—and breaking down those substances with Marker degradation. That's why the "pure" DHEA you buy can be most accurately called semisynthetic.

HUMAN CONVERSION OF YAM EXTRACTS: FACT OR FICTION?

Humans and plants have very different enzyme systems. The fact is that natural plant substances such as diosgenin cannot produce hormones usable by the human body without some laboratory processing.

The clinical data we have that shows DHEA's usefulness is based on known quantities and doses of pure (98 to 99 percent) pharmaceutical-grade material. However, some wild yam extracts and other "precursors" currently on the market are the subject of unsupported claims.

For example, one manufacturer states that using diosgenin or Dioscorea extract enables the body's endocrine system to manufacture its own DHEA. This is impossible. In fact, we know that yam extracts cannot be converted into DHEA, testosterone, progesterone, or any other human steroidal hormone. It is deceptive for a manufacturer or distributor to list the benefits of DHEA and then list their product's content as Dioscorea extract in any amount. There is no correlation between extract concentrations and blood levels of DHEA in humans.

Many people are catching on that the "precursors" or "natural" sources of DHEA do not provide the doses they are looking for. People are now turning to pharmaceutical-grade DHEA, which is being sold in capsules, tablets, sublingual solutions, wax matrices, and oil- and alcohol-based solutions, among other forms.

Always read the manufacturer's or distributor's information very carefully before jumping to conclusions about the potency of a particular form of DHEA. Remember that there is no DHEA per se in diosgenin or yam extracts!

MORE ON THE NATURAL VERSUS SYNTHETIC DEBATE

The natural versus synthetic debate is a highly charged and emotional one in all areas of health and nutrition. People tend to be loaded with emotional attachments to things natural and pure, and manufacturers have long taken advantage of people's emotions through everything from label design to the way the ingredients are listed.

Guarana, for example, is a South American herb containing more caffeine by weight than coffee beans. It produces exactly the same effects and side effects as coffee: a slam to the adrenals and nervous system. But because it's a herb, you'll see it described as "100 Percent Natural Guarana Herb" or similar noninformation.

The same principle has been applied to the labeling of yam extracts, with the result that many consumers have been misled about the true nature of DHEA. Contrary to popular belief, you'll find plenty of evidence that natural is not always better.

What it all comes down to is this: Laboratory-derived substances such as DHEA as well as laboratory-created nutritional supplements have proved both their safety and their effectiveness over many years of use. I challenge you to take a deep breath and give up any preconceived notions you might have about the superiority of purely "natural" substances. Your body will thank you for it.

Other substances that I talk about in this book are also derived from a combination of natural sources and laboratory processes. Take coenzyme Q10, that marvelous bioenergetic nutrient described in Chapter 6. It also is derived from plant raw materials, specifically compounds known as ubiquinones. Yet producing the nutritional supplement known as CoQ10 requires the same combination of natural source and laboratory tweaking as DHEA.

How about another bioenergetic nutrient, AKG—a key element in improving the body's ability to extract oxygen from the air? Its raw material source is also a plant, but obtaining AKG in a usable form requires—you guessed it—laboratory processing.

I know it's a lot to digest. Meanwhile, rest assured that laboratory-derived DHEA has both potency and effectiveness.

99.9 PERCENT PURE?

DHEA can be produced from diosgenin in just a few steps, but don't think you can just mix up a few chemicals and obtain DHEA. Even under the best conditions 100 percent purity of the final product is virtually impossible to obtain.

The issue of purity is becoming more important as more players fight to get on the DHEA bandwagon. If you wish to purchase "pure"

DHEA, you may want to obtain a certificate of analysis (C of A) that states the purity, melting point, and other useful information. However, be aware that this C of A may not mean much, depending on who prepared it, which analytic method was used, and whether the batch number on the C of A matches the actual sample you are buying.

The C of A may be just plain wrong. For example, a DHEA sample obtained from a reliable source that supplies DHEA to pharmacies was found to contain approximately 2.5 percent impurities with structures similar to DHEA and 4 percent impurities with unknown structures that were not steroids. This sample's C of A listed its purity as 99.1 percent.

Discrepancies like these may become a serious problem because unidentified impurities can be toxic. Remember L-tryptophan, which was sold as a sleep aid in health food stores until 1989? Over five thousand cases of a serious blood disorder known as eosinophilia-myalgia syndrome (EMS) and twenty-seven deaths in otherwise healthy individuals were recorded. Eventually all the contaminated L-tryptophan was traced to a single manufacturer, who had used a new, genetically engineered bacterium to make L-tryptophan and had modified the usual purification procedure.

Fortunately, there have been no reported problems related to the production of DHEA. However, it makes sense to exercise caution when taking DHEA if you don't know the source of the product. Look for a manufacturer or distributor that prominently states *on the bottle* (not just in the brochure) that its DHEA is produced using current Good Manufacturing Practices (cGMPs). If enough consumers insist on this type of labeling, it will be adopted by more manufacturers, with tremendous benefits for everyone.

AVOID DHEA ADD-ONS

Some suppliers of pure DHEA combine it with substances such as ephedra (a herbal central nervous system stimulant) and yohimbe (a herb used for sexual impotence). These combinations make no sense at all, except to marketing people motivated by profit margins.

Ephedra (also known as Ma Huang) is a traditional Chinese medicinal herb. Because it stimulates the nervous system much as caf-

feine does, Americans have started using it in large amounts for "energy." However, as with caffeine, it is important to know that ephedra does not provide energy—it just provides stress. Another problem is that there are about forty different species of ephedra, and there is really no way to know which type ends up combined with your DHEA. Certain species contain high amounts of the ephedrine alkaloid, which can raise blood pressure and cause restlessness, headache, dizziness, and irregular heartbeat.

Yohimbine, one of the alkaloids in the herb yohimbe, is available by prescription in the United States, and concentrates of the herb are sold by mail and in health food stores. It can be beneficial in treating sexual impotence when used under the direction of a physician, but many clinicians and the German E Commission (which was set up specifically to evaluate the uses of herbs) do not recommend yohimbe for self-treatment. Touted as aphrodisiacs, yohimbe products can increase blood pressure and cause anxiety or panic—not exactly my idea of a good time.

So if it's DHEA you're after, buy it solo without the dubious "benefits" of other stimulant ingredients.

BIBLIOGRAPHY

Barron RL, Vascoy GJ. Natural products and the athlete: Facts and folklore. *Ann Pharmacother* 1993; 27:607–15.

Ethnobotany and the Search for New Drugs. Ciba Foundation Symposium 185, Fortaleza, Brazil, 30 Nov.–2 Dec. 1993. Wiley, Chichester, UK, 1994.

Lehmann PA. Early history of steroid chemistry in Mexico: The story of three remarkable men. *Steroids* 1992; 57:403–8.

Lehmann PA, Bolivar A, Quintero R. Russell E. Marker: Pioneer of the Mexican steroid industry. *J Chem Ed* 1973; 50:195–9.

Lewis WH, Elvin-Lewis MPF. *Medical Botany: Plants Affecting Man's Health.* Wiley, New York, 1977.

Tausk M. *Organon: The Story of an Unusual Pharmaceutical Company.* Akzo Pharma bv, Oss, the Netherlands, 1984.

Trease GE, Evans WC. *Pharmacognosy,* 11th ed. Bailliere Tindall (Macmillan), London, 1978.

Tyler VE, Brady LR, Robbers JE. *Pharmacognosy,* 8th ed. Lea & Febiger, Philadelphia, 1981.

CHAPTER 11

What Do You Have?
What Do You Need?

Did you hear about the nonswimmer who drowned trying to wade across a stream with an average depth of two feet? Numbers can be deceptive, and that certainly goes for statistics. I've seen enough flaky numbers in my career to fill a barn with a mean cubic volume 200 percent larger than ten bowling alleys laid end to end, running from Chicago to Detroit. You get the picture.

But like it or not, numbers also tell a story, especially when they accurately reflect a specific condition or state of health. You just have to know the *whole* story. People with diabetes have to watch their blood sugar numbers. It's important for you to know your cholesterol level and blood pressure numbers. I encourage you to keep a complete file of all your medical lab results so that you can look back and evaluate trends and changes.

The important point for doctors to remember—an approach taught in medical school but often forgotten—is to treat the person, not the number. This chapter includes charts and numbers regarding DHEA levels, but I want you and your doctor to use them as a guideline, not as a verdict. Medical researchers are always finding people who do not conform to the expectations of charts and projections, for example, people with sky-high cholesterol levels and crystal-clean arteries and people who test positive for the HIV virus but have no signs of immune suppression.

You are a unique individual, and only you and your health care professional can make a clear and accurate determination of the health risk associated with specific DHEA levels. Your physician may opt for the "empirical" approach, which assumes that anyone over age forty has declining levels of DHEA. The doctor will then recommend a prudent dose of 10 to 25 mg and watch to make sure you experience DHEA's benefits without adverse side effects.

I wish it were as simple as consulting a chart and reading a dose recommendation corresponding to a specific test result. Perhaps in the future, when millions of tests have been performed, that will be possible, but right now there's simply not enough data. We do know that different people respond differently to DHEA supplementation. A 25 mg dose in one person may double blood levels, while the same dose in another person may increase blood levels by only 10 percent. The difference might not even relate to DHEA metabolism but instead to differences in digestion, absorption, and even product design.

PRIME PEAK DEFINED

One of the most remarkable things I've noticed in DHEA testing is the wide variability of results within the same age group. One fifty-year-old may have a DHEA level of 200 ng/dl (nanograms per deciliter of blood), while another person the same age may have four times that amount. The only thing we can say with confidence is that people with 800 ng/dl are sending a very good message to their brains: "This organism is healthy and sexually vibrant. Maintain life support and repair at peak levels."

Again, that's because 800 ng/dl is what a twenty- to twenty-five-year-old produces when he or she is at reproductive prime. This *prime peak* level is associated with all sorts of desirable traits, including virility in males and fertility and high libido in females—just the ticket for procreating and ensuring survival of the species.

But Mother Nature doesn't stop there. She knows that having children is an incredible strain on women and that ensuring infant survival requires the continued health of both parents. Thus, prime peak levels of DHEA are also associated with maximum immunity, high metabolic efficiency, and elevated levels of IGF-1, the body's primary repair and rebuild factor. Of course, children (and life in general) also create stress, so high levels of DHEA are also associated with decreased cortisol and enhanced coping skills.

THE TRUTH ABOUT STATISTICS

Benjamin Disraeli once said, "There are three kinds of lies: lies, damned lies, and statistics." Here's what he meant: You see an advertisement for a new diet product in which they tell you that the average weight loss in the clinical trial was twenty pounds in one month. Are you impressed? I hope not.

First, *never put any credence on weight lost in one month.* Everybody loses weight at the start of a diet. The only figures worth reporting are *long-term* figures, at least six months and preferably one to two years.

Second, weight-loss numbers have limited significance unless they are accompanied by equivalent decreases in the percentage of body fat. It is unhealthy and dangerous to lose muscle, but most conventional diets cause a considerable loss of lean muscle tissue.

Third, no good scientist will cite average weight loss because that can be very deceptive. If you request a copy of the clinical report, here's what you are likely to find:

SUBJECT	START WEIGHT	END WEIGHT	CHANGE
1	270	231	−39
2	289	245	−44
3	180	169	−11
4	157	150	− 7
5	149	150	+ 1
		Total weight loss	100 pounds = Average weight loss of 20 pounds for the group

Subjects 1 and 2 were very obese individuals. Just about any type of diet will cause a large amount of water loss in such people, artificially inflating the results. The figures for the other subjects were nothing to get excited about, and in fact subject 5 gained a pound. Still, it is accurate (although not ethical) to say that the group had an average weight loss of twenty pounds in one month.

Are there any factors that would make such a study valid? A larger study group would be a good start. *Average* becomes more meaningful as the data pool increases in size. If, for example, the group contained one hundred people, the weight losses of subjects 1 and 2 would not influence the results as heavily. With five hundred people it would be even less of a factor.

Another approach often used by careful researchers is to remove the highest and lowest scores from each group to eliminate aberrations from the data. Others include the high and low values but make special note of them in what is called the *standard deviation*. When the standard deviation (roughly the average variation within a group) approaches or exceeds the difference between the groups (as in our hypothetical example), the results are said to have *no statistical significance*.

SUMMARY

How can you tell if statistics are reflecting the truth?

1. Check sample size. Large numbers of subjects mean more reliable data.

2. Check "average" results. Regard them with suspicion unless a standard deviation is given.

3. Check scientists. Was the research conducted by competent individuals?

4. Check organizations. Research from the Ozone Center for Intergalactic Studies (and any other unknown sources) should be questioned.

5. Check supporting references. Are the results backed by other published studies?

Obviously, the older you get, the farther you are from prime peak, the lower your DHEA is, and the more worrisome the whole scenario becomes in terms of your adrenal strength and overall health. All indications show that maintaining prime peak levels of DHEA confers significant metabolic benefits, not the least of which may be an increased life span. The converse also appears to be true: Low DHEA levels are linked to a number of killer diseases.

IT'S *YOUR* BLOOD TEST

Every year millions of Americans have an annual physical. They get probed and palpated, screened and viewed, and have routine blood tests. Medicine has made tremendous advances in the last twenty-five years, but these routine blood tests haven't changed a bit. They provide obsolete and in some cases absolutely worthless information, but your doctor orders them every year. Would you like to know why? Because insurance companies pay for it.

In some cases newer and far more valuable tests are readily available, but insurance companies do not want to pay any more than they already are paying. Here's one example: They'll pay for a serum iron level even though the information is meaningless. It only reports how much iron is being transported in your blood, not the level in your tissues. If you complain that this is not an accurate indication of iron status, an insurance company will tell you to look at the complete blood count (CBC), which it will pay for. The idea there is that if you're anemic, you need iron. But you have to be flat-out iron-deficient for about *three years* before you become anemic. Wouldn't it be far better to find out *before* you develop this dangerous and debilitating disorder? Besides, you can have iron levels suboptimal enough to affect your energy level, stamina, immunity, and resistance to cold and still not be anemic. Using anemia to measure iron nutriture is absurd.

A test called *serum ferritin* will accurately and reliably indicate whether you have sufficient iron in your body. It is so accurate that you can use it to determine not only whether you need iron supplements but how much you need. Serum ferritin has been the recognized benchmark for iron nutriture for a decade, but it is not included in any routine blood test. Nearly 50 percent of American women live their entire lives suboptimally nourished in iron, and no one cares to give them the means to correct the problem.

But I digress. Suffice it to say that there are gaping holes in routine blood tests. They measure liver and kidney function (to a degree) and glucose (but not the equally important insulin). They measure cholesterol, but you have to request (and often pay extra for) the really important information concerning the levels of "good" and "bad" cholesterol.

Knowing this, you should not be surprised to find that your insurance company probably will not pay for a DHEA level. After all, those companies have neglected adrenal health for a hundred years. Why change now?

ADRENAL STRENGTH: THE MISSING LINK IN YOUR HEALTH PROFILE

The adrenals produce or contribute to the production of about 150 hormones, every one of which is vitally important to health and wellness. Some manage blood pressure, and others manage stress. And this is all accomplished by two glands no bigger than your thumbs that sit on top of the kidneys.

Chapter 4 presented the scenario of adrenal stress resulting from the strains, burdens, anxieties, and uncertainties of modern life. You saw how this creates a "downward spiral" in which the adrenals become exhausted and problems are then magnified. That occurs because the adrenals are responsible for maintaining *homeostasis* (metabolic and emotional balance) in times of stress. Once that buffer is gone, you are constantly living on the edge of a breakdown.

Imagine living in a constant state of "emergency alert." It would be exhausting. In the same way, these glands, designed for episodes of stress (emergencies) in which tremendous energy is needed to fight or run away from an enemy, find themselves in a situation where this heightened level of activity is required *all the time*. Such is the nature of twentieth-century living. And it's not just job stress. As I explained, it's the pace of modern life and the breakdown of family support groups and community. It's metabolic stress from poor food choices, pollution, and electromagnetic radiation. On top of that, most people add caffeine, a drug that elevates stress hormones and keeps them elevated eighteen hours a day. For the poor adrenals there's just no rest.

It amazes me that more attention has not been paid to the adrenal glands. If you went to your doctor and asked for an adrenal evaluation, he or she would have two tests to administer. One test (for Addison's disease) would tell you if your adrenals were completely shot. The other (for Cushing's syndrome) would tell you if your adrenals were in hyperdrive, most often from an adrenal tumor. Between these two extremes there is nothing your doctor can tell you other than that you appear "normal." Let me remind you that normal is not a state to which you want to aspire.

THE ADVENT OF ADRENOPAUSE

Obviously, there is wide variability in adrenal health aside from Addison's disease and Cushing's syndrome, and I believe that therein lie important secrets regarding energy, stamina, allergy, autoimmune disease, and aging. In fact, the few researchers who recognize this important arena have started to use the term *adrenopause* to refer to the decreased production of DHEA that occurs between the ages of thirty-five and fifty.

Adrenopause is not limited to decreased production of DHEA. We know that DHEA is a parent compound for numerous other hormones and may play a role in scores of other hormonal and non-hormonal reactions throughout the body. Its decline is accompanied by increased risk for cancer, heart disease, stroke, diabetes, osteoporosis, and obesity. Measuring adrenal hormones such as DHEA and cortisol may finally provide a meaningful and sensitive picture of adrenal health.

One West Coast laboratory has developed such a test. Called the Adrenal Stress Index™, this cutting-edge evaluation uses four saliva samples obtained over the course of a day to measure cortisol and DHEA. Then they construct a profile of your adrenal function and give you and your physician concrete information about therapeutic options and follow-up. The test is offered by Diagnos-Techs, Inc., in Kent, Washington (see Appendix A).

EXHAUSTED ADRENALS

The condition known as adrenal insufficiency has been associated with a constellation of symptoms that become more common and severe as we age. They include the following:

Fatigue	Irritability	Depression
Confusion	Anxiety	Inability to concentrate
Insomnia	Cravings for sweets	Headaches
PMS	Indigestion	Poor memory
Rapid heartbeat	Light-headedness	Alcohol intolerance

Conditions known to be associated with adrenal insufficiency include the following:

Allergy	Hay fever	Skin rashes
Asthma	Rheumatoid arthritis	Intolerance to cold

THREE TESTS FOR MEASURING DHEA

Today there are three DHEA tests you can take: serum DHEA, which represents the "free" unbound DHEA in the blood; serum DHEAS, which represents the DHEA bound to sulfate; and salivary DHEA, which represents free DHEA but is measured in saliva instead of blood. Is one of these tests better than the others?

I recommend that your doctor determine which test is best for you on the basis of what you're trying to accomplish. If all you want is a baseline level so that you can monitor the progress of your DHEA Plan, whether it includes supplementation, yoga practice, or deep relaxation tapes, most clinicians recommend serum DHEAS. Here's why.

The stability of DHEA in the blood is such that it is either used up or converted to DHEAS in about thirty minutes. This short half-life makes it useful for measuring inter-day variations of DHEA in response to certain stimuli or time frames, but a more reliable baseline can be obtained by measuring DHEAS, the sulfated form of DHEA, which has a half-life of twelve hours or more. This is a reliable indication of DHEA production because a constant relationship exists between DHEA and DHEAS.

LAB ERROR

No matter which test you select, the benefit you receive from the results depends entirely on their accuracy. Unfortunately, in measuring blood levels of DHEA and DHEAS, much can go wrong. First of all, because these tests are not commonly requested, many labs are not set up to do them. Small labs will often ship the blood to a larger lab. But DHEA blood samples have to be stored and shipped in refrigerated containers, and oftentimes this is not done. Or they may start out in a refrigerated container, but then the container sits in a hot delivery truck all weekend.

Considering the possibility of technician and/or equipment error, it makes sense to deal with a lab that has an industry track record for DHEA testing. Some of these labs are listed in Appendix A. In addition, I would have the blood test performed early in the week, preferably on a Monday or Tuesday, to reduce the risk of transport delays and problems.

Then there are saliva tests, which interest me a great deal because of their convenience and the fact that saliva samples are not as heat-sensitive as are blood samples. Saliva tests have been used for many years to measure other hormones, such as estrogen and cortisol, and I believe there is now a sufficient database to arrive at meaningful numbers for DHEA. Again, it is best to rely on your doctor's experience and judgment to determine which test is best for you.

Advantages of Saliva Tests

1. Saliva tests are less expensive. A single DHEA level from a saliva test costs between $38 and $45. Blood tests commonly cost $55 to $90.

2. Saliva tests are noninvasive. That means no needle in your arm—a significant advantage because the stress of having blood drawn can be enough to invalidate certain blood test results. This can certainly be the case with cortisol, and for this reason salivary measurement of cortisol has been an accepted procedure for years.

3. Saliva levels reflect the free plasma fraction of a hormone.

With DHEA, this is quite valuable because the biological activity of steroid hormones is a function of their free fractions.

4. Saliva tests are convenient. You can even do them yourself at home.

5. Saliva tests make taking multiple samples easy. This is a significant advantage, for example, in measuring the circadian (day/night) fluctuation of a particular hormone.

Disadvantages of Saliva Tests

1. Gum disease can invalidate test results if the saliva is contaminated by blood, artificially raising the DHEA. For this reason the labs listed in Appendix A first perform a test to see if there is any occult (hidden) blood in the saliva sample. Rinsing the mouth with very cold water will often eliminate the contamination problem, and these instructions are included with the sample kit.

2. Most doctors are not familiar with salivary assays. They need to be assured that the information they are receiving is accurate and clinically relevant. The two leaders in the field (see Appendix A) both provide extensive professional support materials as well as trained staff members to answer your doctor's questions both before and after the test is completed.

HOW TO HAVE YOUR DHEA TESTED

If you want a DHEA blood test, you must go to a physician. If you want a DHEA saliva test, there is one lab that will send a test kit directly to your home without a doctor's request (see Appendix A). The problem there, of course, is that you may not be able to interpret the results. In addition, many clinicians like to run a battery of tests along with DHEA, and that makes a great deal of sense.

In a man over age forty, for example, most doctors will want to run a PSA test to measure the risk for prostate cancer. It may be useful for women to have other hormones checked, such as testosterone and the estrogens. Remember that DHEA affects a number of hormones in the body, and there are clinicians who believe that only comprehensive testing can enable you to make intelligent choices regarding a DHEA dose. Working with a physician is the safest and most sensible approach.

WHAT IF YOU DON'T HAVE A DOCTOR?

I suggest calling one of the labs listed in Appendix A. They will be happy to refer you to a doctor in your area who is familiar with DHEA testing. Another approach is to ask around on the Internet or through your network of friends.

ABOUT YOUR TEST RESULTS: NORMAL IS NOWHERE

Whether you choose blood or saliva testing, your results will be reported next to what is called the "reference range," that is, the normal DHEA range for a man or woman your age. If your value falls within these limits, your doctor will naturally tell you that your DHEA levels are normal, at which time your response should be, "Oh no! What can I do?"

Remember that normal people live only seventy-five years, the last twenty of which are typically spent in illness, depression, and chronic pain. The whole idea behind DHEA is to break free from the limitations of evolution and explore the real boundaries of human existence. That means raising your DHEA to prime peak and keeping it there. Once again, in order of importance, here are the factors that will enable you to accomplish that goal:

1. Relaxation and stress revision
2. Optimum diet and regular exercise
3. DHEA supplements if needed

The following chart will give you a clear idea of where your DHEA levels are at the time of testing in relation to prime peak. Remember, the word *normal* in relation to your DHEA levels is irrelevant. You want to do better than that, which is what this book is all about.

MILLIGRAMS, NANOGRAMS, DECILITERS, OR MILLILITERS?

The whole business of measuring DHEA is so new that there is no consensus on how to report test results. Some labs will give you the number of milligrams per deciliter, others will use nanograms per milliliter, and I have seen nanograms per deciliter, milligrams per milliliter, and micrograms per 100 ml. Unless you're a metric weight and volume whiz, you can get a headache trying to see where you stand on the chart.

HOW TO EVALUATE YOUR DHEA TEST RESULTS

1. DHEAS BLOOD TEST

UNIT OF MEASURE		PRIME PEAK	GOOD	DEFICIENT	WORRISOME
mcg/dl	Men	450–600	300–450	125–300	Less than 125
	Women	280–380	150–280	45–150	Less than 45

Note: The unit of measure mcg/dl is the same as mcg/100 ml and μg/dl. If your results are reported in ng/ml (nanograms per milliliter), simply divide the result by 10 and use the above chart to see where you fit in.

2. DHEA BLOOD TEST (FREE, UNBOUND)

UNIT OF MEASURE		PRIME PEAK	GOOD	DEFICIENT	WORRISOME
ng/dl	Men	700–1200	450–700	170–450	Less than 170
	Women	450–800	300–450	120–300	Less than 120
ng/ml	Men	7.00–12.0	4.5–7.0	1.7–4.5	Less than 1.7
	Women	4.5–8.0	3.0–4.5	1.2–3.0	Less than 1.2
mcg/dl	Men	0.7–1.20	0.45–0.7	0.17–0.45	Less than 0.17
	Women	0.45–0.8	0.30–0.45	0.12–0.30	Less than 0.12

3. DHEA SALIVA TEST

UNIT OF MEASURE		PRIME PEAK	GOOD	DEFICIENT	WORRISOME
pg/ml	Men	200–300	100–200	70–100	Less than 70
	Women	125–170	70–125	35–70	Less than 35

Adapted from: Corning Nichols Institute reference values; American Medical Testing Laboratory (AMTL) reference values; Aeron Life Cycles reference values; Michael L. Bennett, Pharm. D.

I believe I have included every possible reporting unit in the charts above. If the charts give you a headache, I understand. We Americans are stuck in the mind-set of ounces, pounds, pints, and quarts, while the rest of the planet uses the far more accurate and workable metric system. If all else fails, ask your doctor or pharmacist for help.

These charts can be used by any adult over age thirty-five. There are no age levels listed on the charts because it doesn't matter what age you are. If you are a mature adult, what you're ultimately trying to do is raise your DHEA levels to prime peak. You'll recall that prime peak levels are the levels of DHEA found in a healthy twenty- to twenty-five-year-old person. That's the level of DHEA you need to trick your body into believing you're young again and to reexperience the physical, emotional, and mental vitality of youth.

OPTIMIZING YOUR DHEA STRATEGY

Say you've consulted your physician and taken a DHEA test. Your test results put you in the "deficient" or "worrisome" range on one of these charts. It's now time to take a good look at your stress (or distress) level. Perhaps you already know that you need some kind of stress revision technique. This is the perfect time to take action.

You reread Chapter 4 and decide to enroll in a yoga class that meets three times a week. Your doctor refers you to a biofeedback trainer, and in a month you feel like a new person. Then you decide to try supplementing with the bioenergetic nutrients described in Chapter 6. Soon you're waking up before the alarm clock goes off, feeling energized and eager to move into the day. You join a walking club with two of your friends, and in a matter of weeks you've lost five of those ten pounds you've been trying to get rid of for years. Now you're ready to retest your DHEA levels, and you find that they've improved significantly, into the "good" range.

Your doctor is pleased because your blood pressure has also gone down. You both agree to explore the possible benefits of raising DHEA to the prime peak range. You start with 15 mg per day. You don't notice anything at first, but then you start feeling more amorous around your husband. You ask for a health club membership for your birthday, and your husband throws in five sessions with a personal trainer. After the first week your trainer remarks that she's never seen anyone progress so well. Sure enough, you can feel the improvements in muscle tone and strength. Everything in your life seems to be getting better, and it couldn't be happening at a better time: Your thirtieth high school reunion is just around the corner.

This is just one possible scenario. With the help of your physician (and Chaper 12 in this book), adapt it as appropriate to your situation. Then get ready to be amazed as these and more astounding results appear in your life.

QUESTIONS AND ANSWERS

Q: At what age should a person start thinking about taking DHEA?

A: There's no reason for anyone under thirty-five to take DHEA unless there's a specific medical need and one is under a doctor's care. After age thirty-five you may want to have a DHEA test to see where you stand.

Q: What about pregnancy and nursing moms?

A. There are no safety studies with pregnant or nursing women. While there is no known toxicity, I recommend that women *not* take DHEA during these times.

Q: When is the best time to take DHEA supplements?

A: Since DHEA levels don't change much throughout the day, it doesn't really matter. If you're taking more than 25 mg, there is some advantage to splitting the dose between morning and evening. Many men report enhanced sexual arousal about 30 minutes after an evening dose.

Q: How do you know the right dose?

A: Health professionals recommend starting with a low dose (5 to 15 mg) and increasing slowly to bring your blood or saliva level to prime peak. I advise everyone to consult a physician, partially because a doctor familiar with DHEA administration will be able to monitor your progress and adjust the dose accordingly. Women usually find that a daily dose in the range of 5 to 25 mg is optimal. Men can often benefit from amounts as high as 75 mg.

Remember that these levels are normal to human metabolism. A twenty-five-year-old man will naturally produce 25 to 50 mg of DHEA per day. By age fifty that amount may be cut by two-thirds. What we are talking about here is a *physiologic* dose, and side effects are rare at this level. Taking much larger doses (in the range of 150 to 300 mg) exceeds the body's normal metabolism. This is known as a *pharmacologic* dose, and you're in no-man's-land at that point. There are physicians who use megadoses for specific therapeutic purposes, but you should *never* do so without professional guidance.

Q: What side effects should I watch out for?

A: In women, too much DHEA can cause acne, irritability, uncomfortable increases in libido, breast tenderness or swelling, menstrual changes, facial hair, and even a deepening of the voice. All these side effects are reversible on discontinuing DHEA.

In men, excessive DHEA also tends to produce acne, and *very* high doses can raise estrogen levels to the point of breast swelling, a condition known as gynecomastia. Signs of hypertestosterone, such as anabolic steroids often produce—aggression, violent outbursts, and irritability—have not been seen with low to moderate doses of DHEA. In both men and women, DHEA supplementation (especially in high doses) may occasionally cause elevations in liver function tests. For this reason, your doctor may want to order these blood tests periodically.

Note: If you have cancer or are at high risk for cancer, be sure to consult your physician before taking DHEA or any other hormone. Some types of cancer, such as prostate cancer in men and ovarian, cervical, or breast cancer in women, are hormone-responsive. In theory, DHEA could accelerate the growth of these cancers.

Q: How long should I stay on DHEA?

A: That depends. If you are enjoying significant benefits, have no side effects, and are staying in the prime peak range, you'll probably want to take DHEA for the rest of your life. If we can extrapolate from animal data, that might be a very long time.

I have been tracking my DHEA levels carefully for eight years, along with a number of other blood tests. After I raised my DHEA to prime peak, my cholesterol went down to 135 and has stayed at that level for five years. My percentage body fat decreased to 9 percent and has stayed at that level with only moderate amounts of exercise. My PSA level (an indication of prostate cancer risk) was low to begin with but has not increased in the last five years. My immune profile has *improved* almost every year, as opposed to the trend among my peers. These are all very good indications of health and wellness. I feel terrific, and I have no intention of stopping DHEA supplementation.

BIBLIOGRAPHY

Aizawa H, Niimura M. Adrenal androgen abnormalities in women with late onset and persistent acne. *Arch Dermatol Res* 1993; 284(8):451–5.

Buster JE, Casson PR, Straughn AB, Dale D, Umsot ES, Chiamori N, Abraham GE. Postmenopausal steroid replacement with micronized dehydroepiandrosterone: Preliminary oral bioavailability and dose proportionality studies. *Am J Obstet Gynecol* 1992; 166:1163–70.

Findlay EM, Morton MS, Gaskell SJ. Identification and quantification of dehydroepiandrosterone sulfate in saliva. *Steroids* 1982; 39:63–71.

Orentreich N, Brind JL, Rizer RL, Vogelman JH. Age changes and sex differences in serum dehydroepiandrosterone sulfate concentration during adulthood. *J Clin Endocrinol Metab* 1984; 59:551–5.

Orentreich N, Brind JL, Vogelman JH, Andres R, Baldwin H. Long term longitudinal measurement of plasma dehydroepiandrosterone sulfate in normal men. *J Clin Endocrinol Metab* 1992: 75:1002–4.

Thomas G, Frenoy M, Legrain, Sebag-Lanoe R, Baulieu EE, Debuire B. Serum dehydroepiandrosterone sulfate levels as an individual marker. *J Clin Endocrinol Metab* 1994; 79:1273–6.

Vining RF, McGinley RA, Symons RG. Hormones in saliva: Mode of entry and consequent implications for clinical interpretation. *Clin Chem* 1983; 1752–6.

Vining RF, McGinley RA. Transport of steroids from blood to saliva, in *Immunoassays of Steroids in Saliva*. GF Reid, D Riad-Fahmy, RF Walker, K Griffiths (eds.). Alpha Omega, Cardiff, CA, 1984, 56–63.

Walton S, Cunliffe W. Clinical, ultrasound and hormonal markers of androgenicity in acne vulgaris. *Br J Dermatol* 1995; 133(2);249–53.

CHAPTER 12

A Day in the Life

The following vignettes are intended to give you a more holistic view of how you can implement the DHEA Plan. They are not prescriptions for you to follow, only examples of what is possible. I want to emphasize again the need to consult a doctor before starting an exercise or supplement program.

The components of the DHEA Plan that will be integrated into these examples are as follows:

1. Food and beverage choices
2. Nutritional supplementation
3. Exercise
4. Stress revision
5. DHEA (testing and possible supplementation)

JANET

Age: Forty-two
Profile: Sedentary office worker
Complaints: Fatigue, overweight, frequent colds, bouts of depression
Goal: To get back in shape, lose fifteen pounds, and feel better

Janet has been burning the candle at both ends by working full time and caring for a ten-year-old daughter and a teenage son. She and her husband are both moderately overweight and haven't exercised consistently for almost ten years.

Janet decided to tackle the coffee issue first. She had seen her use of caffeine escalate to seven or eight cups a day, and she was painfully aware that she was hooked. She tried quitting once, but the splitting headache sent her running back to the coffeepot. This time she took it gradually, decreasing her consumption by one cup a week. At the same time she started taking a bioenergetic nutritional product (see the supplement schedule). When she got down to two cups, she switched to tea, and that worked fine: no headaches, no fatigue.

In fact, after taking the bioenergetics for a few weeks, she noticed that when she arrived home at the end of the day, she didn't collapse on the couch. She started walking with a friend every evening before preparing dinner.

Janet thought she was doing herself a favor by skipping breakfast (and sometimes lunch). She learned that this was only triggering the starvation response, causing her metabolism to drop and fat-storing enzymes to increase. She started having breakfast and even a few healthy snacks throughout the day. With that and a few protein wafers before meals, Janet found that she was eating far less in the evening and didn't crave late-night snacks. Almost without trying, she started to lose about a pound a week; that was nothing to write home about, but it was consistent.

Janet was amazed at how her stress level decreased after she got off coffee. She still had just as much to do, but the constant feeling of struggle, strain, and panic subsided and was replaced by a more patient attitude. Her coworkers all asked what she was taking, and she replied, "Nothing. I'm just off coffee."

The next step for Janet was to see her doctor and have a DHEA test. The doctor prescribed a number of tests and gave her a physical. Based on the test results, Janet started on 10 mg of DHEA a day.

Janet didn't notice anything right away, but after a few weeks she started outpacing her friend on their walks; Janet just wanted to go faster and farther. Although her friend was seven years younger than Janet, she could not keep up. The next month Janet shocked her family by buying a bicycle and announcing that she planned to ride it to work every day.

JANET'S SUPPLEMENT SCHEDULE

(PER DAY)

BIOENERGETICS

Coenzyme Q10	30 mg
Chromium	300 mcg
Alpha-ketoglutaric acid	300 mg
Vitamin B$_6$	15 mg
Ginseng	140 mg

MULTIVITAMIN
One tablet three times a day with food

BONE, CONNECTIVE TISSUE SUPPORT
Two tablets with lunch and two at bedtime
Multi-nutrient formula (see Chapter 6)

ANTIOXIDANT FORMULA
One tablet twice a day

DHEA (10 mg)
One tablet in the morning

She reported to her doctor: "I've got a new lease on life." Increased energy, lost twelve pounds in three months, increased libido, more optimistic, improved sleep, even sense of smell became more acute.

FRANK

Age: Forty-seven

Profile: Aging athlete

Complaints: Fatigue, hypertension, musculoskeletal pain requiring frequent use of analgesics, declining sex drive

Goal: To shake the nagging feeling that "it's all downhill from here"

Frank went to his doctor on fire to get started on DHEA and begin the entire DHEA Plan. Instead, his doctor told him he'd have to take it one step at a time. He was worried about Frank's high blood pressure and family history of heart disease. He didn't want Frank to make radical changes, and he knew next to nothing about DHEA.

The doctor agreed that Frank's diet was superb, and Frank took nutritional supplements on a regular basis. What Frank really needed was help with bone and connective tissue support, so that's where he began with the DHEA Plan. Since he was six feet four inches tall and weighed 256 pounds, he took six tablets a day (three tablets with breakfast and dinner) instead of the four-tablet dose suggested on the bottle.

Frank was amazed to find that in about three weeks he was able to decrease his use of painkillers. Unknown to him or his doctor, the calcium, potassium, and magnesium in the formulation also helped lower his blood pressure, so that on his next visit his doctor decreased the blood pressure medication. That's when everything began to turn around for Frank. One of the side effects of the blood pressure medication was decreased libido, but because Frank was embarrassed about that, he never mentioned it to the doctor. At the new lower dose Frank started getting his sex drive back.

At the same time his stomach pain disappeared. He later found out that was a side effect of the painkillers he'd been taking. Frank was so impressed by these results that he decided to see if he could get off the blood pressure medication altogether. His doctor referred him to a biofeedback therapist, and he started stress revision training. Within a month Frank was off the medication and feeling like a new man.

He continued biofeedback for another month and got so good at it that he ultimately didn't need the machine. He came to know what caused him to become tense and was able to literally "cancel" stress by using the techniques he had learned. When his doctor ordered the saliva DHEA test, it came back right at the prime peak level. There was a note from the laboratory director assuring the doctor that the test was accurate.

Frank was once again amazed. Apparently, getting off painkillers and blood pressure medication, coupled with the biofeedback, was enough to kick his DHEA production up to the level of a twenty-five-year-old. He was elated at the thought of his body starting to rebuild and repair the damage he'd suffered from football injuries, and he decided to see if he could start working out again.

Frank was smart. Even though he was familiar with weights and workout machines, he decided to hire a trainer to make sure he didn't overdo it and help keep his motivation high. His trainer suggested yoga, and Frank just laughed. The thought of twisting his body into a pretzel not only was funny, it was scary. Besides, it would be a waste of time because he could never do those moves, anyway. The trainer assured Frank that the only flexibility required for yoga was an open mind. He told Frank about eighty-year-old clients who benefited tremendously, and that was all Frank needed. If an eighty-year-old could do it, he certainly could.

And he did. From the very first class Frank felt more at ease with his body. He had always had an almost adversarial relationship with his body, pushing it beyond its capabilities and getting angry when it broke down. Now he was moving with a sense of ease, balance, and poise. The yoga postures were strenuous, but he never felt tired afterward. On the contrary, he felt energized for the whole day.

Frank never did start taking DHEA. His levels stayed at prime peak, his joints and tendons got stronger, and his life took a new turn. He decided to take a coaching position at a West Coast university. The last time he was heard from, Frank was into ocean kayaking and Rollerblading.

FRANK'S SUPPLEMENT SCHEDULE

MULTIVITAMIN
One tablet three times a day with food

BONE, CONNECTIVE TISSUE SUPPORT
Three tablets with breakfast and dinner
Multinutrient formula (see Chapter 6)

ANTIOXIDANT FORMULA
One tablet three times a day

He reported to his doctor: "I'm not over the hill—I moved the hill!" Decreased blood pressure, musculoskeletal pain nearly gone, increased energy and libido.

ROBERT AND SALLY

Ages: Robert forty-four, Sally thirty-eight

Profile: Very active, exercise regularly

Complaint: Feel like they lost the "edge" in training and competition

Goal: To win their respective age groups in a national triathlon competition

Robert and Sally were the picture-perfect Florida couple: tanned, muscular, and healthy. But for the last few years, they had been training as hard as ever without getting the results they wanted. Both felt as though the wind had been let out of their sails. They heard other athletes talking about DHEA and decided to give the DHEA Plan a try.

They called a laboratory specializing in hormone testing and were referred to a doctor in their area. The doctor prescribed DHEA blood tests as well as blood chemistries, serum ferritins, a full hormone panel for Sally, and a free testosterone and PSA for Robert. It turned out Sally was iron-deficient. Another doctor had missed that because she was not anemic, but the serum ferritin was clearly below normal. The doctor assured Sally that she'd feel better in a matter of weeks just by taking some iron.

They were surprised to find that their DHEA levels were quite low and that Robert also had low testosterone for a man of forty-four. The lab director informed Robert's doctor that low testosterone is sometimes seen in men who bicycle more than 100 miles a week, possibly as a result of the pressure of the bicycle seat on the perineum. While he was training for an event, it was not unusual for Robert to ride twice that much.

They told the doctor that the only supplement they used was a one-per-day multivitamin and that they even forgot that some days. They each thought that eating "right" would give them everything they needed. The doctor showed them studies indicating that athletes in training have a very difficult time maintaining adequate levels of nutrition and suggested that they follow the DHEA Plan.

They started on the bioenergetics and felt a difference in three days. They felt greater energy in their workouts and recovered more quickly. Robert started with 50 mg of DHEA split between morning and evening. Sally started with 25 mg taken in the morning.

A week later they added a bone and connective tissue support supplement and noticed significant improvement in a matter of weeks. Sally no longer felt the twinges and shooting pain in her shoulder after strength training and for the first time was able to increase her weights to the maximal training level. That gave her a tremendous feeling of accomplishment and boosted her confidence.

Robert began to feel what life was like with adequate testosterone. His problem had been hormonal and nutritional. When both deficiencies were corrected, his performance (on the track and in the bedroom) improved dramatically. Upon retesting, Sally was advised to reduce her DHEA to 15 mg a day and Robert's dose was increased to 100 mg (50 mg in the morning and 50 mg at night).

With optimum nutrition and hormone balance, these two soared. They each came in first in their age groups in a local event and decided to go to Hawaii for the international Ironman competition. To them this was the chance of a lifetime, to see if they could complete the 2.5-mile ocean swim followed immediately by a 112-mile bicycle race and a 26.2-mile marathon.

ROBERT AND SALLY'S SUPPLEMENT SCHEDULE

(PER DAY)

BIOENERGETICS

Coenzyme Q10	40 mg
Chromium	400 mcg
Alpha-ketoglutaric acid	400 mg
Vitamin B_6	20 mg
Ginseng	180 mg

MULTIVITAMIN
One three times a day with food

BONE, CONNECTIVE TISSUE SUPPORT:
Two tablets with lunch, two at bedtime
Multinutrient formula (see Chapter 6)

ANTIOXIDANT FORMULA
One tablet three times a day

DHEA
Sally: 15 mg—One tablet in morning
Robert: 100 mg—50 mg in morning and evening

ADAPTOGENS
Three capsules twice a day
Eleutherococcus (Siberian ginseng) and schizandra

Sally also took extra iron as prescribed by her doctor.

They reported to their doctor: Robert placed fifth in his age group out of five hundred competitors. Sally came in second. Six months later she had to stop taking DHEA because she was pregnant.

EMMA

Age: Seventy-one
Profile: Widow living in a retirement community
Complaints: Adult-onset diabetes, arthritis, obesity
Goal: To be able to travel to her fiftieth college reunion

Emma fell into the downward spiral after her husband died. Used to going for walks with him, she couldn't get motivated to go alone. She stopped cooking and started living on packaged snack foods. If it weren't for Meals on Wheels coming to her apartment once a day, she'd never have had a well-balanced meal.

But she was determined to go to her fiftieth college reunion. Her friends would be there, and more important, college was where she and her husband had fallen in love. At first her desire was dismissed as out of the question by the doctor on duty that day at her HMO, but Emma would not give up. She kept calling until she found a doctor who would help her. In fact, the doctor who agreed to help her had just read a book about DHEA. There was still six months before the reunion, and she thought Emma probably could make it.

She explained to Emma that all her problems were interconnected. Age and obesity caused the insulin resistance that resulted in diabetes. The extra weight and wide fluctuations in insulin caused the arthritis. If they could improve her insulin sensitivity and get her moving, it would be possible to get her on an upward spiral.

In this case the doctor felt that a DHEA test was unnecessary. Emma already had a file two inches thick. She didn't need more blood work, and a saliva test was out of the question because of her bleeding gums. The doctor simply started her on bioenergetics, bone and connective tissue support, and 10 mg of DHEA per day.

A week later the visiting nurse called the doctor to tell her that Emma's blood sugar was low. Interesting, thought the doctor. How could her insulin sensitivity improve that fast? Still, she reduced the dose of Emma's diabetes medicine and talked it over with a colleague. That doctor told her that it was probably related not to the DHEA but to the *chromium* that was in the bioenergetic formula. He explained that chromium is an essential cofactor that works with insulin to regulate blood sugar. Chromium deficiency is quite common in the elderly, and restoring chromium levels can result in significant and rapid improvement in blood sugar control.

Her doctor then found an aquaexercise class for Emma. These classes, often available at community or YMCA facilities, involve movements in a heated pool. The water supports the body and the joints while providing resistance to strengthen muscles. Emma loved it and worked up to attending class three times a week.

Her appetite came back. Unknown to Emma's doctor, this was due to the zinc in the bone support formula. Zinc deficiency is also quite common among the elderly, and one of the first signs of inadequate zinc is loss of taste. This produces a vicious cycle where malnutrition causes loss of taste and loss of taste makes food uninteresting, which contributes to malnutrition. When Emma's taste came back, she started cooking one meal a day, and she actually went to the community cafeteria for breakfast.

In three months Emma lost twenty-seven pounds. Together with daily exercise (she was now using a walker to go up and down the hall on days when she didn't have aquaexercise) and DHEA, this weight loss caused a normalization of her blood sugar. Her muscle tone started to improve, and that also was good for regulating blood sugar. In addition, she was eating regular and sensible meals, not bags of cookies.

Emma did get on an upward spiral. Her weight loss and the bone and joint nutritional support combined to ease her arthritis pain significantly. She started walking without using a cane, and there was a spring in her step whenever she thought of attending her reunion.

She continued to lose weight, primarily because she would not let a day go by without exercise. In addition to her aquaexercise, she was now walking up two flights of stairs instead of taking the elevator. By the time of her reunion, she had lost a total of 45 pounds and felt like a new woman. She even danced a few times with her husband's best friend. Flying back from the weekend, she could only think of all the good things that had occurred in her life, all because of one desire. Now she had a dozen new desires to work on.

EMMA'S SUPPLEMENT SCHEDULE

(PER DAY)

BIOENERGETICS

Coenzyme Q10	30 mg
Chromium	300 mcg
Alpha-ketoglutaric acid	300 mg
Vitamin B_6	15 mg
Ginseng	140 mg

MULTIVITAMIN
One tablet three times a day with food

BONE, CONNECTIVE TISSUE SUPPORT
Two tablets with lunch, two at bedtime
Multinutrient formula (see Chapter 6)

ANTIOXIDANT FORMULA
One tablet once a day

DHEA (10 mg)
One tablet in morning

ADAPTOGENS
One capsule twice a day
Eleutherococcus (Siberian ginseng) and schizandra

She reported to her doctor: "Next comes my seventy-fifth high school reunion!"

YOUR LIFE: SUMMARY GUIDELINES

I've noticed that more and more baby boomers are feeling frustrated with the health movement. They've been told that if they exercise, eat right, and do all the right things (like not smoking, drinking in moderation, etc.), they'll live longer. But this does not appear to be the case. Certainly these lifestyle factors are extremely valuable in reducing risk to catastrophic and degenerative disease, but the boomers are starting to realize that they are aging just like their parents. There is a sense of "Hey, I've been taking handfuls of vitamins every day and doing all kinds of healthy things. Why is my body starting to fall apart?"

If you fall into this category, it's important to know that it's not your fault. You've been doing the best you could with the information available to you. But the truth is that there was a gaping hole in your program, and that was *the hormone factor*. By now, you probably understand it clearly, but it bears repeating: You can eat right, exercise, stand on your head, and drink carrot juice, but none of that will increase longevity as long as your hormones are telling your brain that you're over the hill. It's as if your body is saying, "Why bother?" Until you alter that message, all your other efforts will be in vain.

You now know that you can change that hormone message to: "This body is sexually vibrant, young, and strong. Maintain immunity, brain activity, and repair functions at peak levels." You can reset the ticking evolutionary clock, and send this news to trillions of cells throughout your body. Following are summary guidelines that will help you and your doctor to design a successful optimum health and longevity program.

Remember that chronological age is now obsolete and irrelevant. With the DHEA Plan, it doesn't matter how many candles are on the cake. Your age will be determined by the strength and vitality of your body, the sharpness of your mind, and the passion in your heart. Here's how you can improve those life elements and become younger at any age.

See the Big Picture

Your biological or functional age is determined by many factors, including fitness, immunity, metabolism, the performance of your brain, and myriad biochemical factors. As has been discussed, all of these factors are related to your DHEA level. Thus your primary concern will be maintaining prime peak levels of DHEA. Don't, however, make the mistake of thinking you can just go out and buy a bottle of DHEA. Without attending to the other factors, you will be trying to fill a bucket with holes in it.

Factors that lower DHEA and accelerate aging

- Anything that causes excessive production of stress hormones will lower DHEA. The primary culprits here are stress and caffeine.
- Lack of regular exercise.
- Lack of sleep.
- Adrenal exhaustion.

Factors that increase DHEA and enhance longevity

- Dealing successfully with stress. Deep relaxation.
- Regular exercise, eventually including strength training.
- Mind/body integrating movement such as yoga or tai chi.
- Adequate sleep: experts now believe 8 or 9 hours is optimal.
- DHEA supplementation when necessary.

START YOUR DHEA PLAN NOW, NOT TEN YEARS OR EVEN TEN DAYS FROM NOW

- If you're over thirty-five, start with the bioenergetic and bone and joint support nutrients discussed in chapter 6. Your body needs these raw materials for repair and high-level wellness.
- Sign up for a yoga class. Ultimately, you can follow a video tape,

but in the beginning, you'll need the guidance of a qualified instructor.

- Get a baseline DHEA level (blood test or saliva test), or if you prefer the empiric approach, start taking DHEA according to the following general guideline:

Women:

AGE 35–40: Start with 5 mg, and observe how you feel for a few weeks. Increase to 10 mg if desired after 2 weeks. Review the cautions in Chapter 5.

AGE 40–50: Start with 10 mg. Increase to 20 if desired.

AGE 50–60: Start with 20 mg. Increase to 25 if desired.

AFTER AGE 60: Start with 25 mg. Increase to 50 if desired.

Men:

AGE 35–40: Start with 10 mg, and observe how you feel for a few weeks. Increase to 20 mg if desired after 2 weeks.

AGE 40–50: Start with 25 mg. Increase to 30 if desired.

AGE 50–60: Start with 30 mg. Increase to 50 if desired.

AFTER AGE 60: Start with 50 mg. Increase to 75 if desired.

Conclusion:
Past, Present, and Future

THE PAST

Do you sleep outside on the ground? Neither do I. Most men and women haven't slept on the bare ground for thousands of years, yet our bodies continue to produce earwax, a substance designed to dissuade insects from crawling into our ears when we're asleep. That's just one example of how our bodies are designed to operate in the ancient past. Our DNA hasn't changed in more than twenty thousand years, and back then earwax was really important. Today it's a nuisance.

We've discussed how this time warp of recent human change relates to diet and nutrition—how the human digestive tract is designed for hunting and gathering and the problems that arise from the modern practice of gorging at preset times called meals. Today the only thing most people hunt for is the TV remote.

We're designed for constant exercise and full range-of-motion movement, but today many of us spend hours every day in limited repetitive motion and suffer from joint injuries and carpal tunnel syndrome as a result.

These things are easy to see, but the inner, hidden conflicts between our genes and our behavior are just as real and just as important. To the degree that we can reconcile ourselves to these genetic imperatives, the better our bodies and minds will work. Undoubtedly, the most fundamental of these DNA commands is survival of the fittest. It's what got us this far—the ability of evolution to reward the traits and skills that foster survival. And those skills are not only physical; they are mental and emotional as well.

Not surprisingly, if you look at a group of centenarians, their single most common trait is that they remain *active*. By maintaining physical activity, they continue to send youth messages to their brains, and their brains continue to keep them alive. Their brains *don't know* they're 100 years old.

Aging is not just physical. Elderly people who do crossword puzzles have less degeneration of their brains than do those who sit in front of a television. It's a use-it-or-lose-it world we live in, and crossword puzzles (and a wide variety of other mind-challenging endeavors) keep those neurons firing.

There's also an emotional component of aging. We have discussed the crack-or-cope phenomenon and how those who cope enjoy not only greater health but longer life. Mother Nature is like the coach of a cosmic football team. Just like a college team, new players come along every year, so she is constantly deciding who to keep on the team and who to cut. Which players will she keep on the team? The ones who won't fall apart when the game is on the line.

But it goes way beyond coping. We know that positive feelings of joy, love, and compassion have powerfully positive effects on immunity. You can interpret that in philosophical, religious, or karmic terms, but it's also just plain evolution. Caring for each other is good for the survival of the species. Community builds immunity.

These feelings also correspond to decreases in blood pressure, improvements in sleep patterns, and enhanced brain activation. In fact, joy engages the brain in a much wider spectrum of activity than do even the strongest feelings of anger or fear. We human beings like to feel good, and feeling good has a profound ripple effect throughout the endocrine, immune, cardiovascular, and nervous systems.

Finally, of course, these three areas overlap and accent each other. It's the essential quality of self-esteem, for example, that a "purely" physical accomplishment (winning a race, losing weight, fixing the porch) is accompanied by the emotional and mental feelings of pride and peace.

Even more intriguing is the new awareness of the role hormones play in our experience of life. These biochemicals anchor us to the past because they are the mediators through which change has come. They gave us the strength and stamina to survive in unbelievably harsh times. However, in a way, the stresses of twentieth-century life are worse simply because they are so very *different* and our bodies and minds have not had nearly enough time to adapt.

For over a million years we ate much the same diet, consisting mostly of plant foods, with a significant amount of protein from hunting and fishing. Starchy (sweet) carbohydrates were limited to roots, tubers, and the grasses that predated grains such as wheat.

Today you can go into a convenience store, purchase a 32-ounce soft drink and a doughnut, and deliver to your Paleolithic body more carbohydrates than your ancestors consumed in two weeks. It is the height of folly to assume that we can continue to do this with impunity. In fact, the hormonal response to such metabolic insults is significant and damaging.

The fight-or-flight hormone response gave us superhuman strength to get us out of jams, but the problems we face today do not have teeth and claws. The jams we face are more often traffic jams or paper jams. We do not need the adrenaline rush or the hormonal and nervous system shock to deal with a run in our hose, a nagging boss, the mortgage, a leaky roof, or the puppy mess on the carpet.

DHEA: Nature's Primary Screening Tool

What can we learn from the past that will help us not only to cope but to excel? First of all, Mother Nature (the coach) uses DHEA as her primary screening tool. She uses DHEA to reward the behaviors and activities that support survival and uses the same hormone (by decreasing production) to eliminate those who are no longer an asset to the team.

In youth, DHEA floods our bodies and converts to the sex hormones testosterone and estrogen. But once we are past reproductive age (once we have served our purpose in maintaining species survival), DHEA levels drop steadily. By age seventy-five, the decline in DHEA is approaching fatal. Without adequate DHEA the immune system, cardiovascular system, and brain start to malfunction. Tissue repair ceases, and death soon follows.

With the awareness and technology available to us today, we can finally do something about that. By maintaining prime peak levels of

DHEA we can short-circuit this evolutionary time bomb. Chrono-logical age becomes irrelevant because the message to the brain is now "This organism is healthy and sexually vibrant. Maintain life support and repair at peak levels." With this profound alteration of the aging clock we may be able to enjoy healthy, creative, and disease-free lives of 120 to 150 years.

THE PRESENT

Each facet of the DHEA Plan is essential, and the foundation is stress revision. However, many people view stress revision as the icing on the cake instead of a primary and necessary ingredient in a healthy and successful life. I talk to people all the time who are so busy staying healthy (eating right, exercising regularly) that they have no time to relax. They ask me if I know of anything they could take to help them. "Yes, absolutely," I say. "You can take yoga and meditation. You can take a vacation where you volunteer to help rebuild a Central American village leveled by an earthquake."

DHEA is touted as a stress buster, but that's putting the cart before the horse. Turn that around. Learn to transform stress into a positive force that motivates and inspires you. That way your DHEA levels will rise naturally, sometimes higher than you could accomplish with a pill. Don't forget that you can take a DHEA pill, but if your adrenals are pouring out cortisol (from stress) and your pancreas is pouring out insulin (from excess carbohydrate intake), the DHEA will not last long. It's like trying to fill a bucket with holes in it. Better fix the bucket first.

Developing Perspective

Another important tool is perspective. I arrived home one evening and announced to my wife, "God, I had a terrible day." To which she replied with nothing but compassion, "No, my husband, your wife loves you and your children are safe. You had a great day. These people [pointing to a newspaper article about war in Bosnia] had a terrible day." Perspective often eludes us because we just can't see the big picture. What all the stress revision techniques and pro-grams discussed in Chapter 4 have in common is that they help you to get in touch with your core desires: the things that really matter.

One of the most destructive tendencies of our modern "culture," besides the glorification of violence, is that it takes us away from core desires. Television, magazines, and newspapers implant in our minds a whole set of superficial desires that eventually become compelling. In fact, some people spend an enormous amount of time trying to fulfill those desires, but the promise of materialism is never fulfilled.

Everywhere we turn we are told that if we drive this car, buy that house, land this job, or get that look, we will be happy. Materialism applies not only to things but to people as well. We want to possess people in the same way we want to possess a car or a new house—all with the idea that getting the object will make us happy.

If you're an achiever, able to set goals and work for them, you'll get the job, buy the house, and even marry the person. But somehow getting what you want doesn't provide the sense of lasting fulfillment you long for. In some cases, after struggling to acquire an item, you may even realize that you never really wanted it in the first place. Such is our sorry state of affairs as we get manipulated into all manner of fads and fashions. In reality, it can be said that we are all born princes and princesses and society turns us into frogs.

The danger of a book like this is that people will tend to see DHEA as just something else to "get." It's true that DHEA may give you an additional twenty or thirty years to accumulate more "stuff," but I'm willing to bet you still would not be happy. And I have never seen a hearse pulling a luggage trailer.

A Matter of Focus

Don't get me wrong. I am not saying that possessions are bad; what is unhealthy is the slavelike attachment to them and the belief that they will make you happy. It is literally a matter of focus.

If you have ever taken off in an airplane on an overcast day, you remember the delightful sensation of bursting through the clouds into the brilliant sunlight and crystal blue sky. Similarly, staying above the clouds of materialism dramatically alters our point of view and reveals the vast reality of unconditional joy. Buddhists call this *desirelessness* and remind us that the wealthiest individual is not the one who owns the most but the one who desires the least. I doubt that anyone would disagree with this, yet we spend our lives trying to "get" fulfillment. We are in a way hypnotized by the illusion of materialism.

If this brings to mind images of orange robes, shaved heads, and begging bowls, you've missed the point. Avoiding the trap of materialism does not mean giving up all material possessions. You can, after all, avoid poison ivy without renouncing the entire forest. What is required is *awareness*. When you no longer expect things or other people to provide meaning and happiness in your life, you discover these qualities within yourself. When your attention is no longer "out there" constantly looking for fulfillment, a sense of your own inner power develops, and you experience joy independent of outer circumstances and conditions.

This is an exciting process that I urge you to explore. It is an essential teaching of all the world's religions and the core of yoga, which I consider the science of life. It can be found in what is called the perennial philosophy, the wisdom of the ages, voiced by men and women of vision and insight since the beginning of time. This focus enables us to move beyond evolution into something quite different—something called fulfillment.

Fulfillment is something that nature does not understand. It is purely a development of human consciousness, the unique capacity we have for compassion, understanding, love, and forgiveness. In a way, it is what consciousness develops *after* survival has been assured. It has to do with the quality of life, not just the quantity of life span. We've already discussed the difference between longevity and simply postponing death. Any number of life support technologies can achieve the latter, but true longevity requires a sense of fulfillment.

I am suggesting that fulfillment comes from satisfying core desires, all of which have to do with the precious things in life: friends, families, and commitments in any form to something that transcends material concerns. It's been said in many different ways, but one thing you'll never hear a person saying on his or her deathbed is, "Gee, if only I had spent more time at the office."

This perspective produces what I call "the big relax." It enables us to let go of the harried frenzy that has been foisted on us by a society dedicated only to selling products. By focusing our gaze a little higher, we will see the blue sky and the bright warm sun. Life itself becomes the most valuable gift, and the actions we need to take to find fulfillment finally come into view.

THE FUTURE

Americans have an incredibly wide variety of interests, but eventually we all become gerontologists. That's because, like it or not, we're all in this together and are all growing older. The good part is that our attitudes about aging are changing. Faith Popcorn, one of my favorite social commentators, calls it "down-aging" and notes that "40 is now what 30 used to be, 50 has become like 40, and 65 is the beginning of the second half of life." When she finds out about DHEA, she may revise those numbers upward.

But there are also major challenges to this scenario. In 1996 the first baby boomers turned fifty. In twenty short years they will be seventy, and the number of elderly will grow at an unprecedented rate. No one knows how we will pay for the health care costs of this enormous population. The vast majority of Medicare costs are already incurred by people over sixty-five. But what is more telling is that 9 percent of those elderly people are responsible for 70 percent of total Medicare expenses. That means that even if we succeed in reducing the morbidity of the group as a whole, there will still be astronomical expenses to cover.

We can simply throw money at the problem with more nursing homes, hospital beds, and pharmaceuticals, but who is going to pay for that? A better choice would be to look for ways to keep people healthy as they age. Fortunately, that is starting to happen. After a few false starts, the National Institute on Aging is in full gear, conducting a wide range of research with a 1997 budget of nearly half a billion dollars. Other important work is being done by the National Cancer Institute and other federal agencies.

In terms of developing proactive measures that will work today, I believe this book summarizes the best of what is available. Chapter 6 discussed the value of bioenergetic nutrients and connective tissue support. As you read that material, I hope you were reflecting on how these substances, available in health food stores, could help your parents and grandparents. Remember that remaining active is the key to health, and these nutrients provide the energy, strength, and relief from pain the elderly need to stay active.

Then, of course, there's DHEA. Very promising results have been achieved by giving elderly men and women DHEA supplements of 50 mg per day. Moreover, behavioral therapy to reduce feelings of isolation has resulted in significant increases in DHEA *without supplements*. Clearly, the best results are likely to be obtained with a combination of these approaches. I want to emphasize that consulting a health care professional is imperative. Many elderly individuals are on multiple medications or have limitations that a doctor must evaluate before a safe and effective strategy for DHEA supplementation can be designed.

It's worth the trouble. DHEA, as I have stated, increases IGF-1, one of the body's most important repair-and-rebuild biochemicals. DHEA improves glucose tolerance and helps build muscle. It helps prevent the degeneration of the brain that occurs with aging and, combined with a program to reduce stress, can have a powerful effect on the quality of life for anyone over forty.

The Margin of Health

One of the things that happen to us as we age is that we become increasingly vulnerable to a variety of disease-causing organisms. Much of this is due to decreased immune competence, but there is another side of the equation. I picture what I call the *margin of health* as the difference between immune capacity and total immune stress. Total immune stress, don't forget, includes more than just exposure to bacteria and viruses. Psychological and emotional stress, metabolic imbalances, malnutrition, and "smoldering infections" such as gum disease all add up.

The DHEA Plan is designed to work for people of any age but is particularly appropriate for those over forty. Following the guidelines in this book will accomplish two things. You will decrease total immune stress and at the same time increase your immune capacity. In the following chart you can see that in part A the margin of wellness is very small. Any increase in immune stress (poor sleep two nights in a row) or any decrease in immune capacity (decreased DHEA) will result in illness. In part B, by comparison, there is a very large margin of wellness, and this is how we want to go through life. After all, you don't want to live with the possibility that one mistake (eating too much birthday cake, staying up late) will put you over the edge and make you sick.

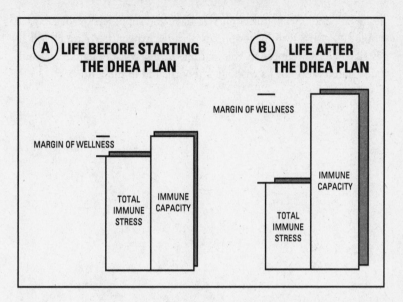

BIOLOGICAL VERSUS CHRONOLOGICAL AGE

How would you like to be twenty years younger? You can do that. I have long believed that measuring age in years is foolish. I prefer to look at biological markers of aging, such as cardiovascular fitness, reaction time, skin thickness, immune strength, organ function, respiratory efficiency, strength, glucose tolerance, and blood pressure. That information gives you what might be called a *biological* or functional age.

The exciting thing about measuring age in this way is that not only is it more accurate, *it can be improved*. Once again, we are making chronological age obsolete by acknowledging that we have the power of choice. We can choose to eat a highly varied natural foods diet. We can choose to exercise regularly and expand that exercise into strength training. We can boost our nutritional intake with supplements and turn back the clock on a number of biological markers. We can choose not to smoke, and we can make efforts to stay focused on core desires.

The wonderful thing about these choices is that they have a very positive impact on those around us: not just the members of our families, who benefit from our vitality, health, and support, but society as a whole. As this awareness spreads, I fully expect it to touch off a renaissance of wellness in this nation. Aging will be feared less and appreciated more for its wisdom, strength, and fulfillment.

Resources

DHEA TESTING LABORATORIES

Blood Testing
Corning Nichols Institute
33608 Ortega Highway
San Juan Capistrano, CA 92690-6130
800-642-4657

American Medical Testing Laboratory (AMTL Corp.)
One Oakwood Boulevard, Suite 130
Hollywood, FL 33020
800-881-2685
954-923-2990

Saliva Testing
Aeron Life Cycles
San Leandro, CA
800-631-7900 or 510-729-0383

Diagnos-Techs, Inc.
6620 So. 192nd Place
Suite J-104
Kent, WA 98032
800-878-3787 or 206-251-0596

RELIABLE SOURCES, INFORMATION ON DHEA, PRODUCT ANALYSIS, AND QUALITY CONTROL

Kaire International Inc.
Leiner Health Products
380 Lashley
Longmont, CO 80501-6048
800-524-7348
FAX: 303-682-9094
http://www.kaireint.com

Advanced Physicians Products
831 State Street
Suite 280
Santa Barbara, CA 93101
800-220-7687
FAX: 800-438-6372

Michael Bennett, Pharm.D.
Xechem, Inc.
908-249-0133
FAX: 908-247-4090
E-mail: mlb @ xechem.com

NEWSLETTERS

Carpe DHEAm: Tools for Life Mastery
Editor: Stephen Cherniske, M.S.
P.O. Box 90331
Santa Barbara, CA 93190-0331
FAX: 805-957-2040
Cutting-edge research on longevity and health
High-tech and high-touch solutions to twentieth-century life
Advanced-technology audio tapes
Subscription: $24 per year

The University of California at Berkeley Wellness Letter
P.O. Box 420148
Palm Coast, FL 32142
Subscription: $24 per year

TOOLS FOR RELAXATION AND STRESS REVISION

The Association for Applied Psychophysiology and
  Biofeedback (AAPB)
10200 W. 44th Avenue, #304
Wheat Ridge, CO 80033
303-422-8436

Institute of HeartMath
P.O. Box 1463
14700 West Park Avenue
Boulder Creek, CA 95006
408-338-8700
FAX 408-338-9861

Preventive Medicine Research Institute
900 Bridgeway #1
Sausalito, CA 94965
800-775-PMRI
415-332-2525

Satchidananda Yoga Ashram
Box 172
Route #1
Buckingham, VA 23921
800-858-9642
804-969-3121

Yoga Journal Video Series
Living Arts
Box 2939
Dept. YJ205
Venice, CA 90291
800-254-8464

CERTIFYING ORGANIZATIONS FOR FITNESS TRAINERS

American College of Sports Medicine
P.O. Box 1440
Indianapolis, IN 46206
317-637-9200

Aerobics and Fitness Association of America
15250 Ventura Boulevard, Suite 310
Sherman Oaks, CA 91403
800-446-2322

IDEA/International Association of Fitness Professionals
6190 Cornerstone Court E., Suite 204
San Diego, CA 92121-3773
800-999-4332

Health Support Organizations

GENERAL HEALTH INFORMATION

National Institute on Aging
(Nat'l Institutes of Health, Health and Human Services Dept.)
9000 Rockville Pike, Building 31, Room 5C35
Bethesda, MD 20892-3100
301-496-1752 for info

National Institutes of Health
(Health and Human Services Dept.)
1 Center Drive, Building 1, Room 126
Bethesda, MD 20892-0148
301-496-2433

ALLERGIES

American Academy of Allergy and Immunology
611 E. Wells Street
Milwaukee, WI 53202
800-822-2762

Asthma and Allergy Foundation of America
1125 15th Street, NW, Suite 502
Washington, DC 20005
800-7ASTHMA

ALZHEIMER'S DISEASE

Alzheimer's Disease Education and Referral Center
P.O. Box 8250-JML
Silver Spring, MD 20907-8250
301-495-3311

Alzheimer's Association, Inc.
919 N. Michigan Avenue, Suite 1000
Chicago, IL 60611-1676
800-272-3900, 312-335-8700 office

The Alzheimer's Foundation
8177 S. Harvard, M/C-114
Tulsa, OK 74137
918-743-0098

ARTHRITIS

National Arthritis and Musculoskeletal and Skin Diseases
Information Clearinghouse
P.O. Box AMS, 9000 Rockville Pike
Bethesda, MD 20892
301-495-4484

CANCER

AMC Cancer Research Center
1600 Pierce Street
Denver, CO 80214
800-525-3777, 303-233-6501

American Cancer Society, Inc.
1599 Clifton Road, N.E.
Atlanta, GA 30329-4251
800-ACS-2345
404-320-3333

American Institute for Cancer Research
1759 R Street, N.W.
Washington, DC 20069
Note: Fabulous newsletter (for a contribution), useful information
and resource guide, great educational material

Bloch Cancer Hot Line
4410 Main Street
Kansas City, MO 64111

Cancer Lifeline
1191 Second Avenue, Suite 680
Seattle, WA 98101
201-451-4542, 800-255-5505 in WA

Cancer Research Institute, Inc.
133 E. 58th Street
New York, NY 10022
212-688-7515

Cancer Support Network
802 E. Jefferson
Bloomington, IL 61701
309-829-2273

Cancer Wellness Center
9701 N. Kenton, Suite 18
Skokie, IL 60079
708-982-9789 hotline, 708-982-9689 office

National Cancer Care Foundation, Inc./Cancer Care, Inc.
1180 Avenue of the Americas
New York, NY 10036
212-221-3300

National Cancer Institute
(Nat'l Institutes of Health, Health and Human Services Dept.)
Cancer Prevention and Control Office
9000 Rockville Pike, Building 31, Room 10A52
Bethesda, MD 20892
301-496-6616 for info

National Cancer Institute
(Nat'l Institutes of Health, Health and Human Services Dept.)
Public Inquiries Office
9000 Rockville Pike
Building 31, Room 10A24
Bethesda, MD 20892
800-4-CANCER, 301-496-5583

CHRONIC PAIN

American Chronic Pain Association, Inc.
P.O. Box 850
Rocklin, CA 95677
916-632-0922

International Pain Foundation
909 N.E. 43rd Street, Suite 306
Seattle, WA 98105

DEPRESSION

Depression and Related Affective
Disorders Association
Johns Hopkins Hospital
600 N. Wolfe Street, Meyer 3-181
Baltimore, MD 21205
410-955-4647

Depression Awareness Recognition and Treatment Program
5600 Fishers Lane
Rm. 1085, Parklawn Bldg.
Rockville, MD 20857
800-421-4211

DIABETES

American Diabetes Association
1660 Duke Street
Alexandria, VA 22314
800-ADA-DISC
703-232-3472

Joslin Diabetes Center, Inc.
One Joslin Place
Boston, MA 02215
617-732-2440

National Diabetes Information Clearinghouse
Box NDIC, 9000 Rockville Pike
Bethesda, MD 20892

EYES

The Lighthouse National Center for Vision and Aging
800 Second Avenue
New York, NY 10017
800-334-5497 TDD, 212-808-5544 TDD

FEMALE HEALTH PROBLEMS

National Women's Health Network
1325 G St., NW
Washington, DC 20005
202-347-1140

HEART AND BLOOD VESSELS

American Heart Association
7320 Greenville Avenue
Dallas, TX 75231-4599
214-373-6300

National Heart, Lung, and Blood Institute
Information Center
P.O. Box 30105
Bethesda, MD 20824-0105
301-951-3260

LUPUS

American Lupus Society
3914 Del Amo Boulevard, #922
Torrance, CA 90503
310-542-8891

Lupus Foundation of America, Inc.
4 Research Place, Suite 180
Rockville, MD 20850
800-558-0121

MALE HEALTH PROBLEMS

Impotence Institute of America
119 S. Ruth Street
Maryville, TN 37801
800-669-1603

The Male Sexual Dysfunction Clinic
4940 Eastern Avenue
Baltimore, MD 21224
410-550-2329

Why Take Vitamin Supplements?

Major diet surveys conducted over the last twenty years have *all* found that large segments of the American population are at risk for suboptimal nutrition.[1-5] The U.S. Department of Agriculture sponsored 178 studies that analyzed the vitamin status of more than twelve thousand people. In summarizing this body of data, Dr. Gordon Graham, a professor of public health at Johns Hopkins University, states: "A large series of surveys carried out in different parts of the country [document] the existence of biochemical and clinical evidence of malnutrition, not limited to our poor, but extending throughout the whole population."[6]

Why is it, then, that when doctors are asked about vitamin supplements, the majority tell you they are unnecessary? Why is it that the same negative response has been issued by the American Dietetic Association, even though surveys show that nearly 60 percent of registered dieticians use supplements themselves?[7]

The answer, unfortunately, has little to do with science or medicine. It is a political and professional issue in which the orthodox medical community and the government have been caught in a catch-22 of their own making. They have, after all, never stated that vitamin supplementation may prove beneficial when administered with knowledge and prudence. Instead, they have repeatedly made the assertion that vitamin supplementation is useless. Now, like the Dutch boy with his finger in the dam, conservative physicians, dietitians, and government health officials find themselves standing against a rising tide of scientific support for nutritional supplementation.

At first there was official denial that anything was wrong with the standard American diet (SAD). Nutritional supplementation was therefore considered unnecessary. After being deluged with research showing major problems associated with the standard American diet,[8] the official position was modified to support widespread dietary change.[9–11]

Today research is published every month that supports not only dietary change but prudent use of nutritional supplements. Studies point to well-defined health benefits, and many speak of nutritional supplements ushering in a "golden age of wellness." This is not an exaggeration. We know from animal and human studies that peak immune function is accomplished only with optimal nutrition.[12,13] With nutrition supplements, this possibility now exists for a great number of people worldwide.

Some practitioners still cling to the irrational contention that nutritional supplements are worthless. Even in the face of overwhelming evidence, many skeptics are waiting for what they consider positive proof. What will it take? *Modern Medicine*, a widely read review journal, ran a lead article entitled "Vitamin Supplements Win New-Found Respect."[14] The piece documented the clear therapeutic benefits associated with supplemental vitamins and minerals and highlighted this statement: "It is a myth that we get all the vitamins we need in our daily diets." Another article in the same issue of *Modern Medicine* presented research showing that a high intake of vitamin C can decrease the risk of heart disease.

Medical World News, a review magazine sent to all members of the American Medical Association, ran a cover story in its January 1993 issue entitled "Vitamins: Emerging as Disease Fighters, Not Just Supplements."[15] *Cardiology World News* (February 1993) highlighted a cover story, "Targeting Atherosclerosis with Vitamins." Also in early 1993, the U.S. Public Health Service started recommending vitamin supplements (containing 400 mcg of folic acid) for the 70 million American women of childbearing age. In 1991 the National Cancer Institute began testing nutritional supplements as anticancer agents, with surprising success. Of course, they didn't call it nutritional therapy but referred to it as "chemoprevention."

Whatever you want to call it, research and clinical support for nutritional supplements is *already* irrefutable. People sitting on the fence with this vital issue should ask themselves two simple questions:

- **DOES NUTRITION AFFECT IMMUNITY?** The answer is undeniably yes. For over a decade worldwide medical literature has been reporting a direct correlation between nutrient status and immune strength.[16]
- **CAN VITAMIN SUPPLEMENTS IMPROVE NUTRIENT STATUS?** Of course they can.[17] No one is saying that vitamins should be used as a *substitute* for a good diet. In fact, studies show that vitamin users generally eat a *better* than average diet and utilize supplements as metabolic "insurance."[18–20] Conservative medicine and government officials say that this isn't necessary, that a well-balanced diet alone can provide adequate nutriture. This simplistic assertion ignores a number of very important facts.

1. NO ONE HAS CLEARLY DEFINED WHAT CONSTITUTES A WELL-BALANCED DIET. Conservative health professionals always refer to the "basic four food groups" to help individuals obtain a well-balanced diet. Unfortunately, this approach is confusing and misleading.

First, combining foods into groups ignores the importance of food *quality*. Someone may well conclude, for example, that ice cream and yogurt are equally nutritious, that cheese offers the same vitamins and minerals as meat, or that a sugared breakfast cereal is as valuable as a slice of whole grain bread. This approach also obscures the importance of variety in the diet. Vegetables and fruits are said to be interchangeable, when in reality these foods contain an entirely different mix of nutrients.

In 1992 the Food Guide Pyramid replaced the "Basic Four Food Group," and although this is an improvement, a number of significant problems still exist. As a concession to the dairy and meat lobbies, for example, the FDA revised the original pyramid designed by top nutritionists. As it exists today, the pyramid actually *recommends* that you consume four to six servings of fatty milk, meat, and eggs every day even though every doctor in the nation knows that those foods promote heart disease and certain types of cancer. Moreover, the pyramid, like the four-food-group circle, offers no clue to food quality. Once again, skim milk and ice cream are grouped together, as are lentils and bologna, olive oil and butter, and whole wheat bread and doughnuts.

Even nutrition texts admit that a diet consisting only of recommended servings from the "basic four" groups is unlikely to provide 100 percent of the RDA of nutrients. One analysis reveals that such a diet would supply only one-tenth to one-half of the RDA for vitamin E, one-half of the RDA for vitamin B_6 and folic acid, and inadequate amounts of thiamine, niacin, vitamin B_{12}, iron, and zinc.[21]

2. FEW PEOPLE ACTUALLY EAT A WELL-BALANCED DIET. Nutritionists agree that to provide all essential nutrients, a diet must be planned intelligently. Careful attention must be paid to the quality of foods selected. Government surveys and independent studies, however, have found that the quality of the standard American diet has been decreasing steadily for over two decades. Analysis of a recent USDA Food Consumption Survey reveals that *none* of the twenty thousand people studied consumed 100 percent of the RDA for all major nutrients.[22]

In 1982 the National Cancer Institute issued guidelines urging the consumption of at least five servings per day from the fruit and vegetable group. This was followed by extensive supermarket promotions and widespread media and public service efforts. Nevertheless, a 1990 survey showed that fewer than 25 percent of California adults consumed five or more fruit and vegetable servings on any day of the week.[23] Nationwide surveys paint a much bleaker picture, with most estimating that only 9 percent of Americans meet this modest dietary requirement.[24]

3. AMONG THOSE WHO DO EAT A WELL-BALANCED DIET, MANY DO NOT DIGEST AND ABSORB AVAILABLE NUTRIENTS. The adage "You are what you eat" is inaccurate at best. In reality, you are what you digest, absorb, and metabolize. Those with poor fat digestion, for example, are at increased risk of vitamin E deficiency no matter how well they eat.[25]

Experts today agree that there are probably millions of Americans suffering from some form of maldigestion and malabsorption. As a consequence, these individuals may be poorly nourished even on a well-balanced diet. Conditions that significantly decrease nutrient absorption include pancreatic, gallbladder, and liver disorders; food allergies; irritation and inflammation of the intestine or colon; surgery on the digestive tract; insufficient acid production in the stomach; low enzyme production; antibiotic therapy; lack of exercise; chronic use of antacids or laxatives; protein deficiency; yeast overgrowth; parasitic infections; and physical or emotional stress. Even the common habit of eating fast and not chewing food well can cause decreased nutrient absorption.

4. THE NUTRIENT CONTENT OF A WELL-BALANCED DIET VARIES WIDELY. A well-balanced diet may not provide textbook levels of vitamins and minerals. Studies have shown that the nutrient content of a food depends on a number of variables, including the climate and soil conditions where it was grown, when it was harvested, how it was shipped, how long and under what conditions it was stored, how it was processed, and, ultimately, how it was cooked.[26–29]

Laboratory analysis of foods from supermarkets across the country revealed that one orange contained 116 mg of vitamin C, while another contained only a trace. One carrot provided 1850 mg of vitamin A, while another contained only 70. One ounce of wheat germ contained 21 mg of vitamin E, another ounce contained only 3.2 mg, and a third was rancid, and all its vitamin E had been destroyed.[30]

5. THE DETERMINATION OF ADEQUATE NUTRITURE IS ITSELF A DEBATABLE CONCEPT. RDAs are established by the Food and Nutrition Board of the National Academy of Science, an organization whose conservative views are often questioned by other medical researchers. The Food and Nutrition Board, for example, claims that 60 mg of vitamin C per day is adequate, yet leading food scientists using careful depletion and replacement procedures have concluded that the intake of vitamin C needed to optimize body stores is *well over twice that amount*.[31]

RDA levels are adequate to prevent vitamin deficiency diseases such as scurvy and beriberi, but very little attention has been paid to conditions that may arise from a *suboptimal* intake of nutrients. For example, many scientific studies in the last ten years have shown a direct relationship between high cancer incidence and lower serum levels of vitamin C, vitamin A, vitamin E, and beta-carotene.[32–37]

Research has also been conducted to compare the frequency of cancer in groups eating a variable but adequate diet. Consistently, these studies show that individuals with the lowest intake of dietary vitamins A, C, E, and beta-carotene have two to six times the risk of certain types of cancer compared with subjects consuming the highest amount of these vitamins.[38–41] Recently, it was reported that high folic acid intake can cut colon cancer risk by one-third.[42] Bio-chemists have even identified numerous mechanisms involved in this anticancer protection.[43,44] It is therefore quite reasonable to say that in many cases cancer is a deficiency disease resulting from suboptimal nutriture.

The same is true for heart disease, the nation's number-one killer. Two recent Harvard University studies that examined a total of 127,000 American adults have shown conclusively that supplementation with high doses of vitamin E can decrease heart disease by 37 percent in men and 41 percent in women.[45,46] The same studies found that a high intake of beta-carotene was associated with a 70 percent reduction in heart disease risk for smokers and a 40 percent reduction among former smokers. Other research shows that vitamin E plays a helper role in this protection.[47]

These are, by anyone's standards, astounding breakthroughs in preventive medicine, so why are physicians not calling up their patients to advise them to utilize these inexpensive and virtually risk-free measures? Because of a pervasive and powerful bias against nutritional supplements. In fact, the Harvard researchers actually caution *against* recommending vitamin E supplementation until more data are available. Astonished at this conclusion, Dr. Dean Ornish, Director of the Preventive Medicine Research Institute at the University of California–San Francisco, stated: "If [these studies] had shown that a drug did this, I don't think they would put that caution in there."[48]

The question of adequacy is also relevant to the study of nutrition and mental development. While it is well established that malnutrition (vitamin deficiency) has a profound impact on mental acuity, very little research has been conducted to evaluate the effect of sub-optimal nutrient intake on child development. Fortunately, studies that have been published support the idea that learning and behavior often are favorably influenced by nutrient intakes beyond RDA levels.[49]

Recommended Dietary Allowances are described as "levels of intake of essential nutrients considered . . . to be adequate to meet the known nutritional needs of practically all healthy persons."[50] The RDA committee admits, however, that these guidelines are not intended to cover needs arising from infections, strenuous exercise, chronic illness, or injury. They also do not take into consideration myriad factors that deplete nutrient stores and/or prevent absorption. When this issue is examined carefully, enormous numbers of people are seen to fall outside the RDA guidelines. For reasons we will now explore, these people can all benefit from vitamin and mineral supplements.

1. INDIVIDUALS TAKING PRESCRIPTION DRUGS. Over 125 million Americans routinely take prescription drugs. Unfortunately, many of these medications interfere with the normal absorption and metabolism of essential nutrients.[51,52] In addition, long-term administration of any prescription drug leads to increased utilization of drug-metabolizing enzymes that can deplete B vitamins such as folic acid.[53]

2. WOMEN USING ORAL CONTRACEPTIVES. Nine million American women use birth control pills, which have been shown to interfere with vitamin, mineral, and amino acid metabolism. Studies show that the long-term use of these drugs can contribute to deficiency of vitamins B_2, B_6, folic acid, and C, as well as magnesium and zinc.[54-56]

3. THE ELDERLY. It is unscientific and absurd to assume that RDAs can be applied to the elderly. Advancing age brings with it myriad changes in activity, digestion, biochemistry, and eating habits. Scientific studies are only now beginning to evaluate these factors, and many are finding that the nutritional requirements of the elderly are actually higher than those of younger adults.[57] At the same time, their nutrient intake is frequently reduced.

Nearly 42 million Americans over sixty-five years of age are therefore at increased risk for malnutrition. Not only do digestion and absorption become less efficient, but elderly people also tend to eat fewer calories and may have problems chewing what they do eat. Low economic status, laxative and diuretic use, and prescription medications can all contribute to malnutrition among this group.[58-60] The *Journal of the American Medical Association* has reported cases of scurvy among elderly men living alone.[61]

Since the elderly segment of society makes the greatest demand on health and social services, many experts believe that nutritional supplementation could be an effective low-cost form of national health insurance. There is more than adequate evidence to support this view.[62-64] Unfortunately, as a result of the prevalent antisupplement bias, public health guidelines regarding supplementation have never been formulated and widespread nutritional testing has not taken place. In fact, much of the literature on supplement use by the elderly has actually been *critical* of the practice. The authors of one survey cite *cost* as a reason for elderly individuals not to use nutritional supplements, even though only 25 percent of those surveyed were supplement users.[65]

The tragedy is that policy makers are influenced by this distorted health care view and, blind to the benefits of prevention, continue to spend billions on high-tech therapies that provide limited benefits. Lamenting this misguided promotion of technology over prevention, an editorial in *Hospital Practice* stated:

> Therapeutic chauvinists fail to recognize that although technologically oriented acute medical treatments (e.g., cardiac bypass, transplants) can have a lifesaving impact for selected patients, they have minimum value in enhancing functional longevity. The greatest advances in health are the result of widely applicable measures to control diseases rather than narrowly applied efforts to reverse the end stages of a disease.[66]

4. THE YOUNG. In an address to the American Academy of Pediatrics, Dr. Lawrence Karlin stated that frank malnutrition is "surprisingly prevalent in certain at-risk groups of children, and in all but the obvious cases goes unnoticed and untreated."[67] His study concluded that children undergoing surgery should have a careful nutritional evaluation, as a marginal nutritional status may increase postoperative complications. He found, for example, that malnourished children had a greater incidence of postoperative infection, required longer intensive care, and were released much later than were adequately nourished children. In fact, of thirty infectious complications in Karlin's study group, twenty-four (80 percent) occurred in the malnourished children.

5. CIGARETTE SMOKERS. There are still over 50 million smokers in the United States whose habit causes, among other things, increased requirements for vitamins C, E, A, and folic acid; the mineral selenium; and perhaps zinc.[68–70] One study revealed that smokers needed about four times the RDA of vitamin C just to maintain adequate serum levels of that essential vitamin. There is even evidence that smokers raise the nutrient requirements of nonsmokers close by, and the Environmental Protection Agency now estimates that "second-hand" smoke kills about 53,000 nonsmokers every year.[71]

6. DRINKERS. Fifteen million alcoholics and roughly 80 million "moderate" drinkers risk malnutrition from alcohol's impairment of nutrient absorption.[72] B-complex vitamins, vitamin C, selenium, magnesium, and the amino acid cysteine all appear to be depleted by excessive alcohol consumption.[73,74] What's more, nutritional therapy has been shown to improve alcoholism recovery significantly.[75]

7. CITY DWELLERS. Roughly two-thirds of the U.S. population lives in major industrial centers where ozone, carbon monoxide, various hydrocarbons, solvents, and other chemical pollutants inflict a significant stress on immunity. A landmark study in the *American Journal of Clinical Nutrition* described the vicious cycle involving environmental toxins and nutrient deficiency.[76] Air and water pollution, occupational exposure to chemical toxins, cigarette smoke, and excessive alcohol consumption all use up massive amounts of protective nutrients. As levels of these nutrients decrease, the body is more seriously damaged by the toxins. Studies suggest that an increased intake of nutrients such as beta-carotene, selenium, vitamin C, vitamin A, folic acid, and vitamin E helps protect against such damage.[77–84]

In addition, toxic metal elements of urban pollution can actually destroy nutrients that are essential for health. Cadmium and lead, for example, have been shown to interfere with the metabolism of zinc, iron, manganese, copper, and selenium.[85,86]

To avoid cadmium and lead poisoning, therefore, scientists have long stressed the importance of maintaining optimal levels of those vital nutrients.[87] Unfortunately, RDA levels for zinc, iron, manganese, and copper do not reflect an increased need for such protection, and the National Academy of Sciences has not established an RDA for selenium.[88]

To make matters worse, independent studies and government surveys consistently show that Americans are *not* getting adequate amounts of these nutrients from a well-balanced diet. Studies have shown that nearly all pregnant women are iron-deficient,[89] and roughly 50 percent of American women will be iron-deficient throughout their entire adult life.[90]

Selenium intake depends almost entirely on the geographic area where food is grown. Although this fact is well recognized, reports in the *Journal of the American Dietetic Association* claim that customary diets "appear" to contain adequate amounts of selenium.[91]

This is a dangerous and unscientific assumption, as illustrated by the fact that the incidence of cancer nationwide correlates directly with the level of selenium in the soil. Where there is a high soil level of selenium, the incidence of cancer is low; in areas where selenium is low, cancer incidence is high.[92] Does this suggest to you that customary diets contain adequate selenium?

What about copper and zinc? In addition to protecting us from lead, mercury, and cadmium toxicity, both minerals are vital to proper immune function.[93,94] One study found that 68 percent of adults surveyed consumed less than two-thirds of the RDA for zinc and 81 percent consumed less than two-thirds of the RDA for copper.[95] This report appeared in the *Journal of the American Dietetic Association*, yet that group still maintains that vitamin and mineral supplements are unnecessary.

8. THOSE SUFFERING FROM CHRONIC ILLNESS. Millions of Americans suffer from recurrent or unrelenting illness. Conditions such as cancer, arthritis, heart disease, diabetes, multiple sclerosis, chronic viral infections, and emphysema may all increase the requirements for specific nutrients.[96,97] Vitamin supplementation therefore can be important in the treatment of these disorders and may accelerate the healing process.[98] In addition, gastrointestinal disorders can dramatically reduce nutrient absorption and appear to be a precipitating factor in serious immune deficiency.[99,100]

Premenstrual tension must be viewed as a chronic health disorder. Surveys indicate that this painful syndrome affects 50 percent of women of childbearing age,[101] and clinical research has shown that many of the symptoms can be relieved through the use of nutritional supplements alone.[102]

Low thyroid function is a commonly overlooked condition, especially in women, and there is much debate about whether routine blood tests are adequate to evaluate this problem.[103] Thyroid hormones help regulate the metabolism of a number of vitamins, and it is not surprising that low thyroid function has been shown to selectively increase nutrient requirements.[104]

9. THOSE SUFFERING FROM ACUTE ILLNESS. Studies show that nutritional status on admission is a good predictor of one's length of stay in the hospital.[105] Those who are optimally nourished heal faster, have fewer complications and infections, and leave earlier. To this day, however, I do not know of a single U.S. hospital that performs routine nutritional evaluations at admission.

During a hospital stay patients are at great risk for malnutrition. The stress of illness, surgery, high fever, and/or extensive burns can create greatly increased requirements for vitamins and minerals.[106,107] It is astounding to note, however, that hospitals do not recognize this fact, as evidenced by the common finding of malnutrition developing *after* admission.[108–111] Some data from U.S. hospitals show a 40 percent rate of malnutrition in inpatient populations and a 60 percent rate in certain surgical patients.[112] This may not seem so surprising in light of other studies showing that many hospitals provide diets that are inadequate *even for healthy persons.*[113]

This may be changing. Research is now showing dramatic benefits from nutritional supplements after surgery. In one study supplemented patients had 70 percent fewer infections, fewer complications, and accelerated recovery compared with controls.[114]

10. ENDURANCE ATHLETES. Although moderate exercise has not been shown to alter nutritional needs, as many as 1.8 million American endurance athletes may have nutritional requirements far beyond RDA levels. Training and competing in endurance sports such as long-distance running, cycling, and swimming appear to cause not only an increased nutrient need but also increased nutrient losses through perspiration, urine, and the rupture of red blood cells in the feet.[115,116] Many experts conclude that such losses, together with an increased metabolic need, cannot possibly be compensated for through diet alone.[117] This conclusion is further supported by studies showing that broad-spectrum nutritional supplementation can improve athletic performance.[118]

11. PEOPLE WHO EAT REFINED OR PROCESSED FOOD. Is there anyone who will disagree with the statement that processed food is the mainstay of the American diet? Does anyone doubt that the processing and refining of food strips away valuable nutrients? I'm amazed to hear normally intelligent people claim that the Standard American Diet provides optimal nutriture. In reality, of course, widespread dependence on processed foods is an irrefutable argument for nutritional supplements.

This is the case because the refining and processing of foods disturbs the entire balance of nutrients. We know, for example, that vitamin A and beta-carotene are insoluble in water and may survive some food processing. However, they are very sensitive to oxidation and are protected only by the presence of vitamin E. When vitamin E is removed or destroyed (a common event), the subsequent loss of vitamin A and beta-carotene may be as high as 90 percent.[119] When beta-carotene is added to margarine, 40 percent of the vitamin is destroyed while it is still being made.[120] By the time the product is shipped, stored, and used, who knows if any of this nutrient is still available?

Virtually all essential nutrients are destroyed to some degree by food processing. The ones that suffer the greatest loss are vitamins C, E, and folic acid, B_6, thiamine, and riboflavin, along with zinc, copper, magnesium, and chromium.

12. PREGNANT AND NURSING WOMEN. Every year over 5 million American women have clearly defined increased nutritional requirements resulting from pregnancy and lactation.[121] Although antisupplement diehards still maintain that such increased needs can be met by diet alone, research does not support their view.[122,123]

In 1991 the issue was put to rest when carefully controlled studies showed that women supplementing with a multivitamin containing 0.4 mg of folic acid were able to decrease their babies' risk of a commonly recurrent birth defect by 72 percent.[124] Subsequent research showed that folic acid could also dramatically decrease the first-time risk for this defect, known as neural tube defect or spina bifida.[125]

Suddenly, instead of physicians being chastised for recommending nutritional supplements, the medical literature was filled with articles and editorials *urging* doctors to put women on vitamins. In September 1992 the U.S. Public Health Service reversed its long-held policy and issued an advisory recommending that all women of childbearing age take a multivitamin containing 0.4 mcg of folic acid.

Neural tube defect is one of the most common types of birth abnormality. Imagine being able to decrease the risk by 60 percent or more simply by taking a multivitamin. Moreover, current research is showing that comprehensive nutritional supplementation (not just folic acid) can reduce the incidence of numerous types of birth defects. In an editorial published in the *New England Journal of Medicine* Dr. Irwin Rosenberg of the Human Nutrition Center at Tufts University observed that there were almost 50 percent fewer birth defects of all types among infants born to women who were given vitamin supplements.[126]

Can you see that the dam is about to break? The amount of research supporting vitamin supplementation is increasing every month, and those holding on to an intractable antisupplement position are starting to look out of touch. What about those who are backpedaling slightly, admitting that perhaps a supplement is a good idea, but not more than the RDAs? This position is also unscientific and absurd.

After all, the RDAs were never meant as guidelines for the formulation of nutritional supplements, and it seems far more reasonable to base supplement doses on current medical literature. In some cases that will call for amounts far greater than RDA levels (e.g., vitamins C and E), and in some cases it will call for less (e.g., vitamin D and iron).

There are many questions regarding the validity of the RDAs. Of paramount importance is the method by which they are determined. The RDA for vitamin E, for example, has been set at 10 mg for men and 8 mg for women.[127] Since vitamin E plays a major role in immunity and cardiovascular health, one might wonder how the Food and Nutrition Board arrived at those numbers.

Did they conduct experiments to determine how much vitamin E is required to adequately protect a person against free radical tissue damage? No. Did they at least carefully evaluate current research relating blood levels of vitamin E and the incidence of cancer, emphysema, heart disease, abnormal blood clotting, and infection? No.

How then did they decide that 10 mg is adequate? The Food and Nutrition Board reviewed several statistical reports and determined that the standard American diet provides from 4 to 10 mg of vitamin E per day. Since they could find "no clinical or biochemical evidence that vitamin E status is inadequate in normal individuals" (the people studied had no distinct deficiency disease), they concluded that this amount must be enough.[128]

It is important to understand how absurd this reasoning is. It literally equates "average" with "adequate," when in fact there is no scientific basis for such a conclusion. For decades Americans were told that it was okay to have blood levels of cholesterol as high as 320 mg/dl. This was within the "normal" range because it was a statistical average for the population. Eventually it was found that blood cholesterol levels over 200 contribute directly to heart disease. In fact, every 5 percent increase over 200 mg/dl increases a person's risk of heart disease by 10 percent.[129]

This means that for decades millions of Americans were at high risk for heart disease without knowing it. It is entirely possible that thousands of these individuals died simply because "average" was considered "ideal."

The same tragic mistake is being repeated today with vitamin E. Ample scientific evidence shows that vitamin E intake two to ten times the RDA can help protect a person against heart disease and cancer.[130–133] USDA scientists have found that immunity can be enhanced by supplemental intake of vitamin E,[134] yet the Food and Nutrition Board continues to maintain that 10 mg (8 mg for women) is adequate and conservative health professionals continue to parrot recommendations for a well-balanced diet. Such folly becomes even more obvious when one realizes that it is based on circular reasoning. They are saying that a "normal" diet provides adequate vitamin E while at the same time defining adequate as the amount provided by a "normal" diet.

ONWARD AND UPWARD

A growing number of health experts are becoming aware that average is not normal, and that normal is not always adequate. Instead of setting nutritional requirements at the quantities necessary to prevent deficiency disease, they are exploring the frontiers of biochemistry to determine the level of intake that will help produce vibrant health.

This represents a fundamental shift from the simplistic and scientifically unreasonable notion that wellness is merely the absence of observable disease. Americans may be adequately nourished in terms of the RDAs, but we are not getting the level of nutrition necessary for disease prevention and maximum longevity.

Recent research has thrown new light on this issue. Experiments with animals tell us that nutrient deficiencies can produce measurable immune defects for up to three generations. In one landmark study mice were fed a diet moderately deficient in zinc. Their offspring appeared normal but exhibited depressed immunity throughout life even though they were fed a normal diet containing adequate zinc. Even more surprising is the finding that the offspring of these normally fed mice also exhibited impaired immune function.[135]

Think about that. This research shows that nutritional deficiencies can carry over for three generations. When you consider the likelihood of multiple nutrient deficiencies in many of our ancestors, it is easy to see how we, the present generation, may experience suboptimal health even while consuming a well-balanced diet. Since we cannot go back and change our grandparents' diet, there is only one prudent course of action. The authors of the above study stated it perfectly: "Perhaps supplementation beyond the levels normally considered adequate may allow for more rapid restoration of immune function."[135]

Breakthroughs in preventive medicine are taking place in research laboratories all over the world. In fact, nutritional immunology is one of the most rapidly expanding areas of medical research today.[136] However, there is a tremendous gap between biochemists and the people who need this information. Fortunately, a growing number of physicians and other health professionals are filling that gap. They risk being branded as mavericks (or worse) by their colleagues, but their vision is clear: Optimum nutrition is the best preventive strategy for reducing pain, suffering, and premature death.

The realm of preventive health care is certainly controversial, but that is the essence of true progress. While the government worries about what is within or beyond the RDA, progressive researchers and clinicians focus on what is safe and effective. While conservative practitioners settle for adequate, most Americans are looking for optimum. In the larger picture it's not that the RDAs are low. Considering the social, genetic, emotional, environmental, and disease factors affecting nutrient status, the RDAs are simply *irrelevant*.

Optimum nutrition strategies can dramatically reduce your risk for all major diseases, including cancer, heart disease, diabetes, and osteoporosis. You can boost your immune strength, conquer anxiety and depression, maximize energy and vitality, and even minimize your risk for diseases thought to be mainly hereditary—all through the power of dietary supplements.

Notes

INTRODUCTION

1. Lardy H, Kneer N, Bellei M, Bobyleva V. Induction of thermogenic enzymes by DHEA and its metabolites. *Ann NY Acad Sci* 1995; 774:171–9.

CHAPTER 2: SEX

1. Sands R, Studd J. Exogenous androgens in postmenopausal women. *Am J Med* 1995; 98(1A):76S–79S

CHAPTER 3: BETTER THAN SEX: STAYING ALIVE

1. Barret-Connor E, Knaw KT, Yen SSC. A prospective study of dehydro-epiandrosterone sulfate, mortality and cardiovascular disease. *N Engl J Med* 1986; 315:1519–24.

2. Araneo B, Dowell T, Woods ML, Daynes R, Judd M, Evans T. DHEAS as an effective vaccine adjutant in elderly humans. Proof-of-principle studies. *Ann NY Acad Sci* 1995; 774:232–47.

3. Spencer NFL, Poynter ME, Hennebold JD, Mu HH, Daynes RA. Does DHEAS restore immune competence in aged animals through its capacity to function as a natural modulator of peroxisome activities? *Ann NY Acad Sci* 1995; 774:200–15.

CHAPTER 4: DHEA, STRESS, AND YOUR LIFE

1. Doc Lew Childre. *Freeze Frame*. Planetary Publications, Boulder Creek, CA, 1994.

CHAPTER 5: DHEA AND WOMEN

1. *All about Fat and Cancer Risk*. American Institute for Cancer Research Information Series, Washington, D.C., 1992, 12.

2. Adlercreutz H. Western diet and Western diseases: Some hormonal and

biochemical mechanisms and associations. *Scand J Clin Lab Investi Suppl* 1990; 201:3–23.

CHAPTER 7: DHEA AND EXERCISE

1. Yen SS, Morales AJ, Khorram O. Replacement of DHEA in aging men and women: Potential remedial effects. *Ann NY Acad Sci* 1995; 774:128–42.

APPENDIX C: WHY TAKE VITAMIN SUPPLEMENTS?

1. First Health and Nutrition Examination Survey (HANES I). 1971–1974. U.S. Dept of Health, Education and Welfare, Public Health Service, National Center for Health Statistics (79-1657), 1979.

2. Ten State Nutrition Survey, 1968–1970. U.S. Dept of Health, Education and Welfare, Health Services and Mental Health Administration, Centers for Disease Control, Atlanta (HSM 72-8130 through 8134), 1972.

3. Nationwide food consumption survey 1977–1978. U.S. Dept of Agriculture, Science and Education Administration.

4. Baker H, et al. Vitamins, total cholesterol and triglycerides in 642 New York City school children. *Am J Clin Nutr* 1967; 20(8):850.

5. National Menu Census 1982. U.S. Department of Health.

6. Fried J. *Vitamin Politics.* Prometheus Books, Buffalo, NY, 1984. 220.

7. Worthington-Roberts B, Breskin M. Supplementation patterns of Washington State dietitians. *J Am Diet Assoc* 1984; 84(7):795–800.

8. An excellent summary can be found in Brewster L, Jacobson MF. *The Changing American Diet.* Center for Science in the Public Interest, 1978.

9. Dietary Goals for the United States. Select Committee on Nutrition and Human Needs, United States Senate, U.S. Government Printing Office, 1977.

10. Diet, Nutrition and Cancer. Committee on Diet, Nutrition and Cancer, Assembly of Life Sciences, National Research Council. National Academy Press, Washington, D.C., 1982.

11. The Surgeon General's Report on Nutrition and Health. U.S. Dept of Health and Human Services, Public Health Service, U.S. Government Printing Office, Washington, D.C., 1988.

12. Chandra RK, Whang S, Au B. Enriched feeding formula and immune responses and outcome after Listeria monocytogenes challenge in mice. *Nutrition* 1992; 8(6):426–9.

13. Good RA, Lorenz E. Nutrition and cellular immunity. *Int J Immunopharmacol* 1992; 14(3):361–6.

14. Kennedy SH. Vitamin supplements win new-found respect. *Mod Med* 1992; 60:15–8.

15. Skerrett PJ. Mighty vitamins. *Med World News* 1993; 34(1):24–32.

16. For an in-depth review of nutrition and immunity, please see the following:

Beisel WR. Single nutrients and immunity. *Am J Clin Nutr* 1982; 35(Suppl):417.

Chandra RK. Immunocompetence is a sensitive and functional barometer of nutritional status. *Acta Paediatr Scand Suppl* 1991; 374:129–32.

Chandra RK. Nutrition, immunity and infection: Present knowledge and future directions. *Lancet* 1983; i:688.

Dreizen S. Nutrition and the immune response—a review. *Int J Vitam Nutr Res* 1979; 49:220.

Gershwin ME, Keen CL, Mareschi JP, Fletcher MP. Trace metal nutrition and the immune response. *Compr Ther* 1991; 17(3):27–34.

Good RA, Lorenz E. Nutrition, immunity, aging and cancer. *Nutr Rev* 1988; 46(2): 62.

Gross RL, Newberne PM. Role of nutrition in immunologic function. *Physiol Rev* 1980; 60:188.

LaVecchia C, Cecarli A, et al. Nutrition and diet in the etiology of endometrial cancer. *Cancer* 1986; 57:1248.

Miller AB, Gori GB, et al. Nutrition and cancer. *Prev Med* 1980; 9:189.

Puri S, Chandra RK. Nutritional regulation of host resistance and predictive value of immunologic tests in assessment of outcome. *Pediatr Clin North Am* 1985; 32(2):499.

Rogers AE, Newberne PM. Nutrition and immunological responses. *Cancer Detect Prevent* 1987; 1(suppl):1–14.

17. Following are a few reports that illustrate that improvements in nutrient status and health can be achieved through appropriate supplementation even in individuals who have no frank vitamin deficiencies.

Cerra FB. Nutrient modulation of inflammatory and immune function. *Am J Sur* 1991; 161(2):230–4.

Cerra FB, Lehmann S, Konstantinides N, et al. Improvement in immune function in ICU patients by enteral nutrition supplemented with arginine, RNA, and menhaden oil is independent of nitrogen balance. *Nutrition* 1991; 7(3):193–9.

Hartz SC, Otradovec CL, McGandy RB, et al. Nutrient supplement use by healthy elderly, *J Am Coll Nutr* 1988; 7(2):119.

Horrobin DF, Campbell A, McEwan CG. Treatment of the sicca syndrome and Sjogren's syndrome with EFA, pyridoxine and vitamin C. *Progr Lipid Res* 1981; 20:253.

Katakity M, Webb JF, Dickerson JWT. Some effects of a food supplement in elderly hospital patients: A longitudinal study. *Hum Nutr Appl Nutr* 1983; 37A:85.

Orwell ES, Weingel RM, et al. Calcium and cholecalciferol: Effects on small supplements in normal men. *Am J Clin Nutr* 1988; 48(1):127.

Stryker WS, Kaplan LA, Stein EA, et al. The relation of diet, cigarette smoking, and alcohol consumption to plasma beta-carotene and alpha-tocopherol levels. *Am J Epidemiol* 1988; 127:283.

Takihara H, Cosentino MJ, Cockett ATK: Effect of low-dose androgen and zinc sulfate on sperm motility and seminal zinc levels in infertile men. *Urology* 1983; 22:160.

Yetiv JZ. Clinical applications of fish oils. *JAMA* 1988; 260(5):665.

18. Kurinij N, Klebanoff MA, Graubard BI. Dietary supplement and food intake in women of childbearing age. *J Natl Diet Assoc* 1986; 86(11):1536.

19. Looker AC, Sempos CT, Johnson CL, Yetley EA. Comparison of dietary intakes and iron status of vitamin-mineral supplement users and nonusers aged 1–19 years. *Am J Clin Nutr* 1987; 46(4):665.

20. Koplan JP, Annest JL, Layde PM, Rubin GL. Nutrient intake and supplementation in the United States (NHANES II). *Am J Public Health* 1986; 76(3):287.

21. Hui YH. *Principles and Issues in Nutrition*. Wadsworth Health Sciences, Monterey, CA, 1985, 305.

22. Crocetti, Guthrie: Eating behavior and associated nutrient quality of diets. Anarem Systems Research Corporation, October 1982.

23. Benefits of fruits, vegetables still go unrealized. *Los Angeles Times*, Aug. 16, 1990, H54.

24. *Nutr Cancer* 1992; 18:1–29.

25. Jeffrey GP, Muller DP, et al. Vitamin E deficiency and its clinical significance in adults with primary biliary cirrhosis and other forms of chronic liver disease. *J Hepatol* 1987; 4(3):307.

26. Schroeder HA. Losses of vitamins and trace minerals resulting from processing and preservation of foods. *Am J Clin Nutr* 1971; 24:562.

27. Nizel AE, Harris RS. The caries-producing effect of similar foods grown in different soil areas. *N Engl J Med* 1951; 244:361.

28. Lappalainen R, Knuuttila M, Salminen R. The concentrations of zinc and manganese in human enamel and dentine related to age and their concentrations in the soil. *Arch Oral Biol* 1981; 26:1.

29. Heffley JD. The role of food supplements. *J Appl Nutr* 1984; 36(2):163.

30. Colgan M. Nutritional requirements of the master athlete. Conference proceedings, Medical and Orthopedic Problems in Sports Medicine, Third Annual U.C. Irvine CME Program on Sports Medicine, Feb. 13–14, 1987.

31. Jacob RA, Skala JH, Omaye ST. Biochemical indices of human vitamin C status. *Am J Clin Nutr* 1987; 46(5):818.

32. LeGardeur BY. Vitamins A, C, and E in relation to lung cancer incidence. *Am J Clin Nutr* 1982; 35:851.

33. Menkes MS, Comstock GW, et al. Serum beta-carotene, vitamins A and E, selenium, and the risk of lung cancer. *N Engl J Med* 1986; 315:1250.

34. Nomura AM, Stemmermann GN, et al. Serum vitamin levels and risk of cancer of specific sites in men of Japanese ancestry in Hawaii. *Cancer Res* 1985; 45:2369.

35. Salonen JT, Salonen R, et al. Risk of cancer in relation to serum con-

centrations of selenium, and vitamins A and E: Matched case-control analysis of prospective data. *Br Med J* 1985; 290:417.

36. Stahelin HB, Rosel F, Buess E, Brubacher G. Cancer, vitamins, and plasma lipids: Prospective Basel study. *JNCI* 1984; 73(6):14673.

37. Wald NJ, Boreham J, Hayward JL, Bulbrook RD. Plasma retinol, beta carotene and vitamin E levels in relation to the future risk of breast cancer. *Br J Cancer* 1984; 49:321.

38. Dietary carotene and the risk of lung cancer. *Nutr Rev* 1982; 40:265.

39. Shekelle RB, Stamler J. Dietary vitamin A and the risk of cancer in the Western Electric study. *Lancet* 1981; ii:1185.

40. Wolf G. Is dietary beta carotene an anti-cancer agent? *Nutr Rev* 1982; 40:257.

41. Bond GG, Thompson FE, Cook RR. Dietary vitamin A and lung cancer: Results of a case-control study among chemical workers. *Nutr Cancer* 1987; 9(2–3):109.

42. Hurley D. High folic acid intake may cut colon cancer risk by one-third. *Med Trib* 1993; 34(12):5.

43. Milner JA. Dietary antioxidants and cancer. *ASDC J Dent Child* 1986; 53(2):140.

44. O'Connor HJ, Habibzedah N, et al. Effect of increased intake of vitamin C on the mutagenic activity of gastric juice and intragastric concentrations of ascorbic acid. *Carcinogenesis* 1985; 6(11):1675.

45. Rimm EB, Stampfer MJ, Ascherio A, et al. Vitamin E consumption and the risk of coronary heart disease in men. *N Engl J Med* 1993; 328(20):1450–6.

46. Stampfer MJ, Hennekens CH, Manson JE, et al. Vitamin E consumption and the risk of coronary disease in women. *N Engl J Med* 1993; 328(20):1444–9.

47. McKeown LA. Vitamin E may cut LDL oxidation. *Med Trib* 1993; 34(8):21.

48. Stolberg S. Studies show vitamin E may reduce heart disease risk. *Los Angeles Times*, May 20, 1993, A21.

49. Colgan M, Colgan L. Do nutrient supplements and dietary changes affect learning and emotional reactions of children with learning difficulties? A controlled series of 16 cases. *Nutr Health* 1984; 3(1–2):69.

50. Committee on Dietary Allowances, Food and Nutrition Board, National Academy of Sciences. *Recommended Dietary Allowances*, 9th ed., 1980.

51. Roe D. *Drug-Induced Nutritional Deficiencies*. AVI Publishing, Westport, CT, 1976.

52. Butterworth CE, Weinsier RL. Malnutrition in hospital patients: Assessment and treatment, in *Modern Nutrition in Health and Disease*. RS Goodhart, ME Shils (eds.). Lea & Febiger, Philadelphia, 1980, 667–84.

53. Parke RJ, Ioannides W. Nutrition in toxicology. *Annu Rev Nutr* 1981; 1:207–34.

54. Fahey PJ, Boltri JM, Monk JS. Key issues in nutrition: Supplementation through adulthood and old age. *Postgrad Med* 1987; 81(6):123.

55. Kishi H, Kishi T, et al. Deficiency of vitamin B6 in women taking oral contraceptive agents. *Res Commun Chem Pathol Pharmacol* 1977; 17:283.

56. Newman LJ, Lopez R, Cole HS, Boria MC, Cooperman LJ. Riboflavin deficiency in women taking oral contraceptive agents. *Am J Clin Nutr* 1978; 31:247.

57. Lowik MRH, van den Berg H, et al. Dose-response relationships regarding vitamin B-6 in elderly people: A nationwide nutritional survey (Dutch Nutritional Surveillance System). *Am J Clin Nutr* 1989; 50:391.

58. Albanese AA, Wein EH. Nutritional problems of the elderly. *Aging* 1980; 7:311.

59. Alford BB, Boyle ML. *Nutrition during the Life Cycle*. Prentice-Hall, Englewood Cliffs, NJ, 1982.

60. Exton-Smith AN: Nutrition in the elderly, in *Nutrition in the Clinical Management of Disease*. Dickerson JWT, Lee HA (eds.). Edward Arnold, London, 1978.

61. Reuler JB, Broudy VC, Cooney TG. Adult scurvy. *JAMA* 1985; 253:805–7.

62. Elmstahl S, Steen B. Hospital nutrition in geriatric long-term care medicine: II. Effects of dietary supplements. *Age Ageing* 1987; 16(2):73.

63. Dunnigan MG, Fraser SA, et al. The prevention of vitamin D deficiency in the elderly. *Scott Med J* 1986; 31(3):144.

64. Newton HM, Schorah CJ, et al. The cause and correction of low blood vitamin C concentrations in the elderly. *Am J Clin Nutr* 1985; 42(4):656.

65. Hale WE, Stewart RB, Cerda JJ, Marks RG, May FE. Use of nutritional supplements in an ambulatory elderly population. *J Am Geriatr Soc* 1982; 30:401–3.

66. Jurivich D, Webster JR. Maimers, killers, and the universal death rate (editorial). *Hosp Prac* 1992; 27(4):12–9.

67. Murray T. Childhood malnutrition may go undetected. *Med Trib* 1993; 35(2):11.

68. Pelletier O. Vitamin C and cigarette smokers. *Ann NY Acad Sci* 1975; 258:156.

69. Schrauzer A. Selenium and cancer: A review. *Bioinorg Chem* 1976; 5:275.

70. Pacht E, et al. Deficiency of vitamin E in the alveolar fluid of cigarette smokers. *J Clin Invest* 1986; 77;789–96.

71. Lesmes GR, Donofrio KH. Passive smoking: The medical and economic issues. *Am J Med* 1992; 93(1A):38S–42S.

72. Shaw S, Lieber CS. Nutrition and alcoholism, in *Modern Nutrition in Health and Disease*. Goodheart RS, Shils ME (eds.). Lea & Febiger, Philadelphia, 1980.

73. Sprince H. Protectants against acetaldehyde toxicity: Sulfhydryl compounds and ascorbic acid. *Fed Proc* 1974; 33(3):1.

74. Peters R. The case for vitamin-fortified booze? *Food Product Dev*, Sept. 1980.

75. Biery JR, Williford JH Jr, McMullen EA. Alcohol craving in rehabilitation: Assessment of nutrition therapy. *J Am Diet Assoc* 1991; 91(4):463–6.

76. Thomson A, Jeyasingham M, Pratt O. Possible role of toxins in nutritional deficiency. *Am J Clin Nutr* 1987; 45:1351.

77. Brin, M. Drugs and environmental chemicals in relation to vitamin needs, in *Nutrition and Drug Interrelations*. Hathcock JN, Coon J (eds.). Academic Press, New York, 1978.

78. Shamberger RJ, Willis CE. Selenium distribution and human cancer mortality. *Crit Rev Clin Chem* 1971; 2:211.

79. Menkes M, Comstock G, Vuilleumier J, et al. Serum beta-carotene, vitamins A and E, selenium, and the risk of lung cancer. *N Engl J Med* 1986; 315:1250–4.

80. Kawai-Kobayashi K, Yoshida A. Effect of dietary ascorbic acid and vitamin E on metabolic changes in rats and guinea pigs exposed to PCB. *J Nutr* 1986; 116(1):98.

81. Burton GW, Ingold KU. Beta carotene: An unusual type of lipid antioxidant. *Science* 1984; 224:569.

82. Goodman DS. Vitamin A and retinoids in health and disease. *N Engl J Med* 1984;310:1023.

83. Parke RJ, Ioannides W. Nutrition in toxicology. *Annu Rev Nutr* 1981; 1:207.

84. Basu TK, Schorah CJ. *Vitamin C in Health and Disease*. AVI Publishing, Westport, CT, 1982.

85. Spivey MR, et al. Micronutrient interactions: Vitamins, minerals and hazardous elements. *Ann NY Acad Sci* 1980; 355:249.

86. Kutsky RJ. Selenium: Ascorbic acid, in *Handbook of Vitamins, Minerals and Hormones*, 2d ed. Kutsky RJ (ed.). New York, Van Nostrand Reinhold, 1981.

87. Demopoulos H, et al. Cancer in New Jersey and other complex urban/industrial areas. *J Environ Pathol Toxicol* 1980; 3(4):219.

88. Food and Nutrition Board. Recommended Dietary Allowances. 10th rev. ed. National Academy of Sciences, Washington, D.C., 1989.

89. Fairbanks VF, et al. (eds.). *Clinical Disorders of Iron Metabolism*, 2d ed. Grune & Stratton, New York, 1971.

90. Sturgeon P, Shoden A. *Am J Clin Nutr* 1975; 24:469.

91. Watson RR, Leonard TK. Selenium and vitamins A, E, and C: Nutrients with cancer prevention properties. *J Am Diet Assoc* 1986; 86(4):505.

92. Shamberger RJ. Relationship of selenium to cancer: I. Inhibitory effect of selenium on carcinogenesis. *JNCI* 1970; 44(4):931.

93. Prasad AS. Clinical, endocrinological and biochemical effects of zinc deficiency. *Clin Endocrinol Metab* 1985; 14(3):567.

94. Sorenson J. Therapeutic uses of copper, in *Copper in the Environment*, *Part II*. Wiley, New York, 1979.

95. Holden JM, Wolf WR, Mertz W. Zinc and copper in self-selected diets. *J Am Diet Assoc* 1979; 75:23.

96. Chandra RK. Nutrition, immunity, and infection: Present knowledge and future directions. *Lancet* 1983; i:688.

97. Dodge JA. The nutritional state and nutrition. *Acta Paediatr Scand* 1985; 317:31.

98. Goldberg P, Fleming MC, Picard EH. Multiple sclerosis: Decreased relapse rate through dietary supplementation with calcium, magnesium and vitamin D. *Med Hypotheses* 1986; 21(2):193.

99. Archer DL, Glinsmann WH. Intestinal infection and malnutrition initiate acquired immune deficiency syndrome (AIDS). *Nutr Res* 1985; 5:132.

100. MacDermott RP. Cell-mediated immunity in gastrointestinal disease. *Hum Pathol* 1986; 17(3):219.

101. Hargrove JT, Abraham GE. The incidence of premenstrual tension in the gynecologic clinic. *J Reprod Med* 1982; 27:721.

102. Stewart A. Clinical and biochemical effects of nutritional supplementation on the premenstrual syndrome. *J Reprod Med* 1987; 32(6):435.

103. Barnes BO, Galton L. *Hypothyroidism: The Unsuspected Illness.* Crowell, New York, 1976.

104. Cimino JA, et al. Riboflavin metabolism in the hypothyroid human adult. *Proc Soc Exp Biol Med* 1987; 184:151.

105. Robuck JT, Fleetwood JB. Nutritional support of the patient with cancer. *Focus Crit Care* 1992, 19(2):129–30, 132–4, 136–8.

106. Whitney EN, Cataldo CB, *Understanding Normal and Clinical Nutrition.* West, St. Paul, 1983.

107. Blackburn G. Nutrition assessment in clinical practice. *Postgrad Med* 1982; 71(5):46.

108. Bollet AJ, Owens S. *Am J Clin Nutr* 1973; 26:931.

109. Bistrian BR, et al. *JAMA* 1974; 230:85.

110. Dempsey D, Oberlander J, et al. Vitamin deficiencies in general surgical patients. *Surg Forum* 1983; 34:84.

111. Lemoine A, LeDevehat C, et al. Vitamin B1, B2, B6, and C status in hospital patients. *Am J Clin Nutr* 1980; 33:2595.

112. Murray T. Childhood malnutrition may go undetected. *Med Trib* 1993; 35(2):11.

113. Butterworth CE. *JAMA* 1974; 230:879.

114. Daly JM, et al. Supplemented enteral diet boosts postoperative surgical outcome. *Surgery* 1992; 112(1):56–67.

115. Hiller WDB, O'Toole ML, Massimino FA, et al. Plasma electrolyte and glucose changes during the Hawaiian Ironman Triathlon. *Med Sci Sports Exerc* 1985; 17:219.

116. Falfetti HL, Burke ER, et al. Hematological variables after endurance

running with hard and soft soled running shoes. *Physician Sports Med* 1983; 11:118.

117. Crosby LO. Substrate utilization, body composition, and nutrient requirements in endurance athletes. *Ann Sports Med* 1987; 3(2):104.

118. Colgan M. Nutritional requirements of the master athlete: Preventive maintenance and performance enhancement. Conference proceedings, Medical and Orthopedic Problems in Sports Medicine, Third Annual U.C. Irvine CME Program on Sports Medicine, Feb. 13–14, 1987.

119. De Ritter E. Stability characteristics of vitamins in processed foods. *Food Technol* 1976; 30:48–54.

120. Marusich W, De Ritter E, Bauernfeind JC. Provitamin A activity and stability of beta carotene in margarine. *J Am Oil Chem Soc* 1959; 34:217.

121. Williams SR. *Essentials of Nutrition and Diet Therapy.* Mosby, St. Louis, 1982, 179–83.

122. Taper L, Oliva JT, Ritchey SJ. Zinc and copper retention during pregnancy: The adequacy of prenatal diets with and without dietary supplementation. *Am J Clin Nutr* 1985; 41:1184.

123. Zamorano AF, Arnalich F, et al. Levels of iron, vitamin B12, folic acid and their binding proteins during pregnancy. *Acta Haematol* 1985; 74(2):92.

124. MRC Vitamin Study Research Group. Prevention of neural tube defects: Results of the Medical Research Council Vitamin Study. *Lancet* 1991; 338:131–7.

125. Werler MM, Shapiro S, Mitchell AA. Periconceptual folic acid exposure and risk of occurrent neural tube defects. *JAMA* 1993; 269(10):1257–61.

126. *N Engl J Med* 1992; 327:1875–6.

127. Food and Nutrition Board, National Research Council. *Recommended Dietary Allowances,* 10th ed. National Academy Press, New York, 1989.

128. Food and Nutrition Board, National Academy of Sciences. RDA Monograph on Vitamin E. U.S. Government Printing Office, 1974.

129. Sherwin R, Kaelber CT, et al. The Multiple Risk Factor Intervention Trial (MRFIT): II. The development of the protocol. *Prev Med* 1981; 10:402.

130. Gey K, Brubacher G, Stahelin H. Plasma levels of antioxidant vitamins in relation to ischemic heart disease and cancer. *Am J Clin Nutr* 1987; 45:1368.

131. Menkes MS, et al. Serum beta-carotene, vitamins A and E, selenium, and the risk of lung cancer. *N Engl J Med* 1986; 315(20):1250.

132. McKeowne-Eysses G, Holloway C, et al. A randomized trial of vitamin C and vitamin E supplementation in the prevention of recurrence of colorectal polyps. *Prev Med* 1987; 16:275.

133. Beisel W. Single nutrients and immunity. *Am J Clin Nutr* 1982; 35:416.

134. Maugh TH. Vitamin E can boost immunity, study finds. *Los Angeles Times,* Sept. 30, 1988, 3.

135. Beach RS, Gershwin ME, Hurley LS. Persistent immunological consequences of gestation zinc deprivation. *Am J Clin Nutr* 1983; 38:579–90.

136. Beisel WR. History of nutritional immunology: Introduction and overview. *J Nutr* 1992; 122(Suppl 3):591–6.

Glossary

Acetylcholine—a chemical produced by the brain and nervous system that transmits nerve impulses.

ACTH—(adrenocorticotropic hormone, also called corticotropin and adrenocorticotropin)—a pituitary hormone that acts on the adrenal glands, stimulating their growth and the production of steroids such as epinephrine, cortisol, DHEA, and other corticosteroids. Its production is increased during times of stress.

Adaptogen—a substance that helps buffer the stress response, making the body more resilient to tension, anxiety, or physical strain.

Adrenal—an endocrine gland that lies above each kidney.

Aerobic—an organism or metabolic process that requires oxygen.

Aldosterone—a steroid hormone that regulates water and electrolyte balance.

Allergen—a substance that causes an allergic reaction, more properly called an antigen.

Allergenic—capable of producing an allergic reaction.

Alzheimer's disease—a progressive condition in which nerve cells in the brain degenerate. Symptoms include forgetfulness, memory loss, disorientation, dysphasia (loss of speech coordination), anxiety, mood changes, and confusion.

Anabolic—the phase of metabolism in which living tissue is built up and maintained; the constructive phase of metabolism.

Analogue—a compound that is structurally similar to another compound.

Androgens—hormones, including testosterone, DHEA, DHEAS, and androstenedione, that promote male characteristics. Women also produce androgens, but they are overshadowed by the estrogens.

Antibody—a protein produced by the immune system in response to any foreign substance (antigen) such as a virus or bacterium.

Antigen—any substance that precipitates an immune system reaction with an antibody. Bacteria, viruses, pollen, dust, mold, and incompletely digested food are common antigens.

Antioxidant—a substance that protects the body against damaging free radicals. Different antioxidants protect the body in different ways. Some prevent free radicals from forming. Others neutralize free radicals once they are formed. Still others enhance the body's ability to repair free radical damage. The best known antioxidants are vitamins C and E, beta carotene, coenzyme Q10, and the mineral selenium.

Autoimmune—immune system activity directed at normal body tissues. Examples include rheumatoid arthritis, lupus, and multiple sclerosis.

Bioenergetic nutrients—a group of essential nutrients involved in the body's production of energy, including coenzyme Q10, alpha-ketoglutaric acid, the B-complex vitamins (especially B6), aspartic acid, creatine, and the mineral chromium.

Biofeedback—a stress management technique that uses an electronic device to measure minute changes in the tension level of the body and/or brain. Visual or auditory "feedback" instructs the mind as to which thought patterns cause stress and relaxation so that the individual learns to defuse potential stressors before they affect the adrenal and cardiovascular systems. This training takes place on the subconscious as well as the conscious level of awareness.

Boron—a trace mineral important in the maintenance of bone and connective tissue. Also involved in the synthesis of certain hormones, including estrogen and testosterone.

Catabolic—the phase of metabolism in which energy is made available via the breakdown of molecules; the destructive phase of metabolism.

Catalyst—a substance that changes (usually accelerates) the rate of a chemical reaction without itself undergoing a change. Many enzymes are catalysts, but not all catalysts are enzymes. Cata-

lysts are always specific for a particular process and cannot be interchanged.

Cell membrane—another name for the cell wall, made up primarily of fatty acids.

Cholesterol—a fatlike steroid alcohol made by the liver or absorbed from the diet. It is needed to make bile and is important in the synthesis of steroid hormones.

Choline—a B-complex vitamin found in both meat and vegetables; also synthetically produced. Helps keep fat from depositing in the liver. One form of choline, acetylcholine, is essential for nerve function.

Chondroitin sulfate—one of the primary mucopolysaccharides; an important constituent of cartilage, tendons, and ligaments (see *mucopolysaccharides*).

Chromium—an essential trace mineral that plays a cofactor role with insulin in glucose metabolism.

Coenzyme Q—the collective name for a group of biochemical substances called ubiquinones, which perform coenzyme functions like a vitamin, behave like an enzyme, and resemble fats. A numerical designation (from 6 to 10) is added to the name, depending on the molecular structure. The most common ubiquinone found in the human body is coenzyme Q10 (CoQ10).

Control group—provides a standard to compare and evaluate experimental observations. A control group is identical to an experimental group except for the one factor being studied.

Corticosteroid—any steroid (including glucocorticoids) produced by the adrenal cortex.

Cortisol—a glucocorticoid that comes from the adrenal cortex. Pharmaceutically it is called hydrocortisone.

Diosgenin—a substance commonly derived from the Mexican wild yam. In a laboratory diosgenin can be altered to produce a number of steroids, including pregnenolone (the precursor to DHEA) and progesterone. Claims have been made that ingesting diosgenin will raise serum levels of DHEA, but it is not possible for the body to make this conversion. Diosgenin may, however, provide other health benefits.

Duodenum—the upper portion of the small intestine (about 12 inches) that leads from the stomach to the jejunum. A great deal of the

digestive process occurs in the duodenum, along with most
nutrient absorption.

Endocrine—having to do with glands that secrete hormones and other
chemical messengers into the bloodstream. The adrenals, pineal,
hypothalamus, thymus, pituitary, pancreas, testes, ovaries, and
thyroid are all endocrine glands.

Endogenous—any substance produced within a cell or organism. The
opposite of *exogenous*.

Epidemiology—the study of disease distribution among selected groups
or populations. An epidemiologist is a scientist specializing in
epidemiology.

Epinephrine—a hormone produced mainly by the adrenal glands but
also manufactured in the brain and nervous system. The product
name is Adrenalin. Epinephrine is the chief stress or emergency
hormone, causing increases in heart rate and respiration and
having profound effects on the blood vessels, muscles, and brain.

Estrogens—hormones, including estrone, estradiol, and estriol, that
promote female characteristics. Men also produce estrogens, but
they are overshadowed by the androgens.

Excipient—a nonnutritive substance added to tablets or capsules. Some
excipients (such as microcrystalline cellulose) are added to help
tablets disintegrate. Others are used to facilitate manufacturing,
such as the vegetable stearates that help bind ingredients together
and prevent tablets from sticking to the press.

Exogenous—any substance supplied from outside an organism. The
opposite of *endogenous*.

Fat-soluble vitamins—vitamins A, D, E, and K, which do not dissolve in
water but are absorbed, transported, and stored as part of a molecule of fat. Fat-soluble vitamins differ from water-soluble vitamins
in that they are stored in fairly large quantity in the body, primarily in the liver and fatty tissue.

Fatty acids—a straight-chain monocarboxylic acid that is a component
of fat. Fatty acids are classified as saturated (no double bonds
within the molecule), monounsaturated (one double bond in the
molecule), and polyunsaturated (multiple double bonds within
the molecule). Essential fatty acids cannot be made by the body
and must be obtained through diet. These include linoleic acid,
perhaps gamma-linolenic acid, and arachidonic acid.

FDA—The U.S. Food and Drug Administration.

Free radical—an unstable and dangerous molecular fragment with an unpaired electron. Free radicals are highly reactive substances produced by normal metabolism and used as part of the body's immune arsenal. Such free radical reactions, however, are carefully regulated by other substances and enzymes called free radical scavengers or antioxidants. Unfortunately, free radicals are also produced by radiation, industrial pollution, and the peroxidation breakdown of fats. Such free radical exposure may exceed the body's control mechanisms, and damage can occur as the radical tries to restabilize itself by stealing available electrons from surrounding tissue. It is believed that such free radical damage contributes to a wide range of disorders, including heart disease and cancer.

GABA—(gamma-aminobutyric acid)—a biochemical produced in the brain that inhibits brain neurotransmitters.

Ginseng—a tonic or medicinal herb that has been shown to assist in the cellular production of energy, although it is not classified as a stimulant. Siberian ginseng, also known as Eleutherococcus, has more of an adaptogen effect, assisting the body to handle stress. A variety of ginseng roots have been used in traditional Asian medicine for centuries.

Glucocorticoids—hormones that affect carbohydrate metabolism by promoting glucogenesis (creation of glycogen by the liver) and raising blood sugar levels. Glucocorticoids also influence fat and protein metabolism, increase muscle tension, help maintain arterial blood pressure, inhibit inflammatory and allergic responses, decrease the circulation of immune cells in the blood, cause lymphatic tissue to shrink, and stimulate many functions of the central nervous system.

Gonad—a testicle or ovary.

GRAS—a classification used by the FDA to indicate that a substance is generally recognized *as* safe; also referred to as the GRAS list. Absence from the GRAS list does not necessarily mean that a substance is unsafe, only that its safety has not been determined.

Hormone—a chemical substance that regulates the activity of certain organs or a specific organ.

Hypothalamus—a gland located deep within the brain that controls part of the pituitary gland by secreting vasopressin, oxytocin, and other hormones. The hypothalamus plays a role in mood, appetite, and functions of the hormonal and autonomic nervous systems.

Insulin—a hormone secreted by the pancreas that regulates blood sugar levels.

Interferon—a type of cytokine, specifically a glycoprotein, that kills viruses by inhibiting the creation of viral RNA and proteins. There are three types of interferons: alpha, beta, and gamma. All animal cells are able to produce interferons.

Interleukin—a group of cytokines produced by the immune system in response to antigenic or mitogenic stimulation. Some interleukins are used for the treatment of solid malignant tumors.

In vitro—occurring under external laboratory conditions, such as in a test tube.

Immunosenescence—age-related decline in immunity.

In vivo—occurring within a living organism.

Lipid—the chemical or medical name for fats and oils.

Libido—the desire for sexual activity.

Lymphocyte—a small cell found in the blood, lymph, and lymphoid tissues. Part of the body's immune system, these cells grow, differentiate, and become activated when they come in contact with antigens.

Macrophage—a large immune cell originating as a monocyte in bone marrow. Macrophages usually can't move until stimulated by inflammation. When activated they engulf foreign particles and other microorganisms. Their immune function also includes the secretion of enzymes.

Metabolism—the physical and chemical process by which living tissue is built up and maintained and energy is made available via the breakdown of molecules. These two phases of metabolism, the constructive phase (called anabolism) and a destructive phase (called catabolism), together build up and feed the body.

Microbe—any microscopic organism, including viruses and bacteria. Commonly called "germs."

Molecule—a group of atoms joined by chemical bonds. The term also refers to the smallest possible amount of a substance that maintains its individual characteristics.

Monocyte—an immune cell that is formed in the bone marrow and lives in the blood for about 24 hours. After 24 hours, a monocyte migrates to various organs and develops into a macrophage.

Mucopolysaccharides—a group of polysaccharides that, when combined with water, form an essential component of mucus and connective tissue.

Natural killer cell—a specialized immune cell with particular anticancer and antiviral capabilities.

Neuron—a highly specialized nerve cell that can be stimulated and can conduct impulses.

Neurotransmitter—a substance that leaves the axial end of a neuron and travels to another neuron, stimulating it. Messages are relayed throughout the body this way. Examples of neurotransmitters are acetylcholine and norepinephrine.

Norepinephrine—both a neurotransmitter and a neurohormone, it is a vasoconstrictor, elevates blood pressure, and increases the heart rate.

Pathogen—any microbe or agent that causes a disease.

Peroxisome—a microbody that can be found primarily in kidney and liver cells and contains enzymes such as amino acid oxidase, catalase, and urate oxidase. It functions to break down the products of oxidation within the tissues.

Phagocyte—a cell with the ability to engulf foreign particles and other microorganisms (the action is called phagocytosis).

Pituitary gland—an endocrine gland located at the base of the brain that stores and secretes numerous important hormones that contribute to a wide variety of bodily functions.

Pheromones—substances similar to hormones that are secreted along with perspiration and perceived by another member of the same species, producing a change in the sexual or social behavior of the perceiver.

Placebo—an inert substance such as cornstarch, sugar, or sterile water that is given as medication under the guise of being a real drug. A placebo can have a positive effect, a negative effect, or no effect on the recipient. Placebos are often used on the control group in clinical trials to factor out results that are not due to true physiological effects but arise from the "placebo effect" or expectations of the recipient.

Platelet—a tiny disk- or platelike structure. The most common type is the blood platelets. Blood platelets affect the clotting and coagulation of blood. They also take up, store, transport, and release the hormone serotonin.

Precursor—something that precedes or acts as a building block for another substance.

Pregnenolone—a steroid hormone that is a precursor to progesterone and DHEA.

Prostate—a gland in males that surrounds the urethra and neck of the bladder. It secretes a milky fluid that combines with sperm to form semen.

Receptor—a molecule that lies on the surface or inside a cell and recognizes and binds with specific molecules, fitting with them like puzzle pieces. The activated receptor causes a change within the cell. A receptor can also be a sensory nerve ending, which responds to stimuli.

Senescence—the process of aging.

Serotonin—a neurotransmitter and hormone that causes vasoconstriction, stimulates smooth muscle, and influences mood and memory.

Sterol—any steroid, such as cholesterol. Sterols are fat-soluble.

Testosterone—the most potent male sex hormone (androgen), secreted primarily by the testes. Testosterone stimulates the development of male reproductive organs and male sex characteristics, such as the beard. It encourages bone and muscle development.

Thymus—a ductless gland located beneath the upper part of the sternum. Having an immune system function from fetal life on, it reaches maximum development during puberty, and its size and function decline with age.

Index

acquired immune deficiency syndrome (AIDS), 7–8, 51, 58–59, 218
adaptogens, 81, 208, 241, 244
adrenal glands, 20, 24, 36, 59
  and prime peaks of DHEA, 222
  strength of, 223–25
  stress and, 77, 83–84, 223–24
  weight management and, 155–57
  women and, 98–99, 108
adrenopause, 224
alcohol, 100, 103, 176, 187, 192, 200, 275
alignment principle, 109–10
allergies, 83–84, 203–4, 224
alpha-ketoglutaric acid (AKG), 114, 116, 118, 166, 207, 215
androstenedione, 31–32
anemia, 222, 239
antibodies, 59–60, 63, 65–66, 201
asthma, 62
atherosclerosis, 5, 7, 44, 46, 115, 191, 198
autoimmune disorders, 50, 64–65, 83, 98, 188, 224
awareness factor, 13–14

Banting, F. G., 210
B cells, 51, 65

behavior, 6, 15, 29–30, 38, 41, 63, 77–78, 82, 109, 173, 205
bench flies, 145
Best, Charles H., 210
bioenergetics, 30, 112–19, 215, 253
  availability of, 118
  benefits from, 119
  exercise and, 113–14, 116–17, 133–34, 139–40
  nutrition and, 30, 113–18, 207
  stress and, 87–90
  super six in, 113–16
  upward spiral with, 116
  and vignettes on implementing DHEA Plan, 235–36, 239–40, 242–43
  vitality self-evaluation and, 116–17
  weight management and, 113, 115, 117–18, 166, 183
blood pressure, 16, 230, 255
  adrenal strength and, 223
  nutrition and, 191, 198, 208
  past and, 248
  stress and, 75–77, 79–80, 83
  survival and, 43–44
  and vignettes on implementing DHEA Plan, 236–37
  weight management and, 156

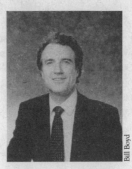

Bill Boyd

About the Author

STEPHEN CHERNISKE, M.S., is a leading biochemist and medical writer, an early DHEA researcher, and one of the first scientists to personally take DHEA and quantify the results. He is a trained nutritionist, a college instructor in clinical and sports nutrition, and a popular lecturer. Mr. Cherniske is author or coauthor of four books on health and nutrition, and numerous articles in popular and scientific publications. He is a member of the National Academy of Research Biochemists, the American Medical Writers Association, and the Editorial Advisory Board of *Ms. Fitness* magazine. Stephen Cherniske lives with his wife and two young sons in Santa Barbara, California.